DOUBLE PLAY

Training and Nutrition Advice from the World's Experts in Baseball

Bob Alejo, CSCS
Jose Antonio, PhD, CSCS, FISSN
Bill Campbell, PhD, CSCS, FISSN

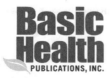

Basic
Health
PUBLICATIONS, INC.

The information contained in this book is based upon the research and personal and professional experiences of the authors. It is not intended as a substitute for consulting with your physician or other healthcare provider. Any attempt to diagnose and treat an illness should be done under the direction of a healthcare professional.

The publisher does not advocate the use of any particular healthcare protocol but believes the information in this book should be available to the public. The publisher and authors are not responsible for any adverse effects or consequences resulting from the use of the suggestions, preparations, or procedures discussed in this book. Should the reader have any questions concerning the appropriateness of any procedures or preparation mentioned, the authors and the publisher strongly suggest consulting a professional healthcare advisor.

Basic Health Publications, Inc.
28812 Top of the World Drive
Laguna Beach, CA 92651
949-715-7327 • www.basichealthpub.com

Library of Congress Cataloging-in-Publication Data

Alejo, Bob.
    Double play : training and nutrition advice from the world's experts in baseball / Bob Alejo, Jose Antonio, Bill Campbell.
        p. cm.
    Includes bibliographical references and index.
    ISBN 978-1-59120-180-9
    1. Baseball—Training. 2. Athletes—Nutrition. I. Antonio, Jose, PhD.
II. Campbell, Bill (William) PhD. III. Title.

    GV875.6.A57   2008
    613.7'11—dc22

                                                    2008006996

Editor: John Anderson • Copyeditor: Jon VanZile
Typesetting/Book design: Gary A. Rosenberg • Cover design: Mike Stromberg

Printed in the United States of America

10   9   8   7   6   5   4   3   2   1

Contents

Introduction

Why Baseball
Needs This Book

Roughly 12 million people play baseball in the United States. Add to that the baseball-crazy countries of Japan, the Dominican Republic, and other Caribbean countries and you have one of the few truly global sports. You might even include softball because the same basic principles of training and nutrition also apply there. But this book isn't about how to play baseball—it is about how to get your body in better shape to play the best baseball of your life. Eating right, taking the right supplements, and engaging in a periodical and proper training regimen all contribute to your overall baseball performance.

In this book, we'll demolish common myths associated with training and nutrition for baseball. For instance, it is a total myth that weight training will ruin a good swing or a good pitching arm. In fact, there could not be anything further from the truth. Weight training can add more power to a swing and produce a healthier, stronger arm! Also, you'll find out if pitchers should lift weights. We know hitters are weight-room junkies, but what about pitchers? A complete weight-lifting program for baseball players is provided in the book.

We also touch on the many conditioning methods used in the baseball world. Many coaches have little, if any, understanding of the energy sources used while playing. Let's just say this: running around a track as if you're a cross-country runner is nothing less than an ignorant approach to baseball training. It's a great way to make you a *slower* baseball player.

Without spending too much time on the science behind aerobic and anaerobic metabolism and training, let's define those energy sources from a commonsense perspective. Aerobic metabolism is oxygen dependent and uses sugar and fat as primary fuels. The least powerful of all the energy systems (something to keep in mind while training), aerobic metabolism supplies the fuel for continuous, rhythmic exercise performed by large muscle masses over extended periods of time, as in jogging, distance swimming, or bicycling. Anaerobic metabolism occurs in the absence of oxygen and is a short-lived source of energy—it is the most powerful of the energy systems. Highly anaerobic movements, such as weightlifting, take two minutes or less before exhaustion. Intensity is the determining factor as to which energy source is used and for how long. For instance, if you can maintain a movement for twenty minutes or more, then the intensity level must be low to very low. Likewise, you can imagine what kind of intensity is needed to "burn out" in less than two minutes.

Now that we have defined both major energy sources, we can look at the game and evaluate if activity levels are high or low and come to a conclusion as to baseball's primary energy source. It becomes clear that anaerobic pathways fuel baseball movement, so conditioning of an anaerobic nature best simulates the demands of baseball activity, better preparing the athlete and reducing the risk of injury.

Simply put, long-distance running, or thirty to forty minutes of continuous cardiovascular work, is a poor way to condition a baseball athlete and might even slow progress.

Then there is the issue of speed. In essence, speed kills—or, rather, lack of it will help you get "killed" by the opposing team! Whoever said you couldn't improve speed is wrong. Granted, each of us has a certain speed potential, but very few athletes ever reach their full potential. This means that nearly every athlete can improve his speed, especially baseball players. Why? Because baseball speed is not dependent on straight-ahead speed. Baseball speed is seldom needed over long distances, and it's not simply about running fast. You can learn techniques for speed development. All things being equal, a faster ballplayer is certainly a better ballplayer. Sample workout regimens for off-season, preseason, and in-season are provided.

And, of course, we touch on the importance of healthy eating and the controversial subject of sports supplementation. Because baseball is essentially a speed/power sport, the dietary needs of baseball players more closely resemble those of weight lifters than distance runners. For instance, there is no need for baseball players to consume large amounts of carbohydrates, as they do not expend the amount of energy seen with typical endurance athletes. Instead, baseball players should focus on eating unprocessed carbohydrates, lean proteins (fatty fish, which is a great, high-fat source of protein, should be consumed regularly), and unsaturated fats.

Regarding supplements, baseball players can benefit from several nutrients that might help improve mental acuity, speed recovery, and produce gains in lean body mass. For instance, there is exciting new research on leucine and other essential amino acids. Leucine supplementation has been shown to increase upper body power. Also, even though vitamins do not directly provide energy or increase muscle mass, they do support normal energy metabolism. The best sources of vitamins are fruits and vegetables, and we repeatedly recommend throughout this book that athletes eat these types of foods every day. That being said, in reality, few individuals eat perfectly every day. For this reason, we recommend that you take a quality multivitamin with minerals.

It's time to get away from the old-school (and wrong-school) approach to nutrition and training for baseball and embrace the latest scientific advances from the leading experts. With this book, we will provide you (and your coaches) with the tools for making yourself the best baseball player you can be.

1

The Ultimate Baseball Athlete

Those in charge of physical training often design and implement programs that are far too advanced or "cutting edge" for their target athletes. Lengthy lists of fancy, complex, and, at times, senseless exercises that contribute little to true strength or power are becoming the rule instead of the exception. Also, to suggest there are some exercises that baseball players should not perform is unproven. The bottom line is this: If basic strength is not achieved by basic movements, then an athlete will not reach his or her full strength or power-producing potential.

"SPORT SPECIFIC"

Let's touch on an important but often misused term: "sport specific." By definition, sport specific implies that a comprehensive training program should result in an increase in physical qualities associated with a specific sport, thus enabling better performance. A comprehensive program has several components, all of which, when integrated, result in the desired outcome. Many trainers have claimed to have designed sport-specific baseball weight-training programs. In reality, it would be difficult in many of these programs to find any exercise that looks like baseball! The exercises in a truly comprehensive program should strengthen muscles that, when combined with a well-designed conditioning and skill-improvement program (practice), leads to improvement in performance.

In other words, there are no sport-specific exercises but rather *exercises that train sport-specific muscles*. For example, the bench press does not simulate any baseball movement, but since upper body strength is important for baseball players and the bench press stresses a large muscle mass, plus a few smaller ones and shoulder stabilizers, the bench press becomes sport specific for baseball.

The game of baseball is played with the entire body. No one swing or throw comes from any one muscle—the whole body is generating movement to create power or speed. To think that a program that solely emphasizes forearm strength and rotational exercises will improve performance is to think that the world is flat. Even though some muscles or movements are more dominant than others, the entire body has to be effectively strengthened in order for you to be the best player possible. Properly strengthened and conditioned muscles produce better results and allow other muscles (antagonists and stabilizers) to work more efficiently. As an example, a stronger upper back allows the front of the shoulder girdle to work with less stress and effort, reducing the chance for injury and improving throwing strength and endurance.

A balanced weight-training program is critical to performance and injury prevention. If a program overemphasizes any area of the body, not only is there a better chance of being injured, there might also be a loss of strength, power, and sometimes flexibility. In a sport that inherently emphasizes one-sided throwing and swinging, imbalances are big issues. So, while it is important to train rotational abdominal strength to simulate throws and swings, additional training for the lower back and opposite-side movements (left-handed movements for right-handers and vice versa) must be included for balance.

A SCIENTIFICALLY BASED EXERCISE PROGRAM

There is little support for the idea that baseball athletes should not perform certain exercises. There is such an enormous volume of strength and conditioning research that to base a decision on this type of uneducated guess is careless. A few widely held concepts that may seem logical but also prove to be myths upon further research include: overhead pressing is bad for the throwing shoulder; touching the chest while bench pressing will tighten the chest and ruin the arm for throwing; and heavy squatting is bad for the knees.

Now, for those with a past or present history of shoulder limitations or injuries, overhead pressing and limited range-of-motion chest pressing might be prescribed in some or all phases of training. But this restriction is for *all* athletes with symptomatic shoulders, not just baseball players. Certainly, any athlete or nonathlete should take precautions when squatting if there is a past or present knee injury. However, research indicates that squatting can further strengthen a healthy knee and improve a limited or injured knee. The point is that a scientific and evidence-based training and conditioning program with clear objectives and strategies will provide the baseball athlete with the best opportunity to become physically prepared.

COMPONENTS OF A BALANCED PROGRAM

Although this book focuses on strength training, conditioning, and nutrition, several other components play an important role in developing baseball's best athlete. Flexibility training (stretching), comprehensive warm-ups, cross-training as an alternative to traditional conditioning, and the use of restorative measures (e.g., whirlpools, massages, rehabilitation) must be planned for or added when necessary if an athlete is to reach the highest level.

Stretching and warm-up exercises of varying intensity should be performed prior to all physical activity. While the stretching program should basically remain unchanged, the warm-up should be directly related to the activity. For example, prior to running, the warm-up would include mostly running drills (backpedals, high knees, skipping, etc.). An upper body weight-training day would begin with arm swings and stretches and medicine ball work.

There are times when injury or limitation makes it impossible to run. This is not restricted to lower body injury: many shoulder, upper back, and elbow injuries prohibit a player from running. During those times, it is important to continue training without aggravating the injured or limited parts by substituting stair-stepper, bicycle, treadmill, or elliptical machines. Lastly, staying healthy includes having a certified athletic trainer or physician evaluate aches and pains to prevent lost playing time or serious injury. Additionally, massages and hydrotherapy (whirlpools, showers) have been proven to speed recovery and healing from intense training or competition.

Strength Training

What is the purpose of increasing strength? Will it make you a better baseball player? Yes, it will, if you are able to transfer the strength you have into baseball-specific activities. More accurately, strength is the root of all that is good. It is the foundation for speed, power, and endurance. This section will discuss what it takes to make you the strongest player you can be.

Obviously, the goal of resistance training—in this case, weights are the resistance—is to increase your strength, but as an athlete (especially a baseball player), strength training is much more than just getting stronger. *One of the most important benefits of strength training often goes unnoticed: reducing the risk of injury.* So, preventing injury through the right kind of training program is as important as gaining strength. Exercises chosen for the targeted muscles are important for two reasons: optimally training those muscles is necessary to perform at the highest levels, and it is also critical to improve or maintain a healthy athlete.

Conditioning: What Fuels Baseball's Fire?

Many conditioning methods used in the baseball world continue to prove there is little, if any, understanding of the energy sources used while playing. Without spending too much time on the science behind aerobic and anaerobic metabolism and training, let's define those energy sources from a common-sense perspective. Aerobic metabolism is oxygen dependent and uses sugar and fat as primary fuels. The least powerful of all the energy systems (something to keep in mind while training players), aerobic metabolism supplies the fuel for continuous, rhythmic exercise performed by large muscle masses over extended periods of time, such as jogging, distance swimming, or bicycling. Quite the opposite, anaerobic metabolism (there are two types) occurs in the absence of oxygen and is a short-lived source of energy. It is the more powerful of the energy systems. Highly anaerobic movements, such as weight lifting, can only be performed for two minutes or less before exhaustion. It is plain to see that intensity is the determining factor as to which energy source is used and for how long. For instance, if you can maintain a movement for twenty minutes or more, the intensity level must be low to very low. Likewise, you can imagine what kind of intensity is needed to "burn out" in less than two minutes.

Now that we have defined both major energy sources used for work, we can look at the game and evaluate if activity levels are high or low and then determine baseball's primary energy source. Someone unfamiliar with baseball could watch a game and easily come to the conclusion that baseball is not that tough on the body and not tiring at all. Even the most ardent fan might rate the fitness level of some players as poor. While it is true that some players have average fitness levels, it requires peak fitness to perform at the highest level. Why, if there is little activity in a three-hour game, does a player need to be in top shape to perform? Because when activity does occur—fielding a ground ball hit to the outfield, base-running, pitching, hitting—it is dynamic, requiring appropriate levels of strength and even higher levels of conditioning for performance and injury prevention.

And considering the length of a baseball season (up to seven months at the professional level), there is little doubt that players need to be in great shape. Furthermore, game action is not continuous but intermittent, involving powerful bursts of speed and usually requiring all-out effort. So, even though the seasons are long, addressing short-term strength and effort through anaerobic training better prepares the athlete and also provides season-long endurance.

In summary, comparing the two energy sources reveals completely opposite modes and effects. Considering that game-like movements are forceful, it makes sense to condition in the same manner. While aerobic energy provides fuel for low intensity activity and extended periods of time, it does not prepare an athlete for the type of endurance necessary for aggressive, intermittent baseball movement. Anaerobic pathways fuel baseball movement, and conditioning of an anaerobic nature best simulates the demands of baseball activity, better preparing the athlete and improving the necessary physical qualities that reduce the risk of injury. Simple long-distance running or 30–40 minutes of continuous cardiovascular work is a poor way to condition a baseball athlete and might even slow progress.

Flexibility Training

Flexibility training is usually dominated by a stretching program. However, flexibility is also improved by special warm-up drills, full range-of-motion resistance training, and many conditioning, agility, and coordination drills. We recommend a stretching routine with two components: dynamic and static flexibility. Typically, static exercises begin the flexibility session, followed by the dynamic movements just prior to activity (games or practices).

Static stretching exercises are what most people think of as stretching. An example of a static stretch is to sit on the ground with the legs straight and reach for your toes, thereby stretching your hamstring muscles. These stretches are held for 15–30 seconds. Dynamic exercises include jogging in place and touching your heels to your buttocks, exaggerated high-knee running, or walking lunges with intermittent jumping.

THE MAJOR MUSCLES USED BY BASEBALL ATHLETES

Before determining what training program is best, you need to understand the muscles used when performing basic baseball skills such as swinging, throwing, fielding, and running. Different baseball skills share the same movement patterns, thus sharing the same muscles. For example, throwing and swinging are ground-based rotational patterns that rely heavily on the lower back, abdominals, and obliques. Leg strength is equally important in providing support for the body, maximizing ground reaction forces, and allowing for maximum torque production from the trunk. Conversely, there are some muscles that are not commonly shared yet are critical to baseball. In particular, the rotator cuff is arguably the most important musculature for throwing but not a necessity for fielding or hitting.

Again, while it is not necessary to be an expert in anatomy, programs are often wrongly designed as a result of a misunderstanding or a lack of knowledge in regard to baseball-related movements. Let's take a look at these fundamental movements and the major musculature involved.

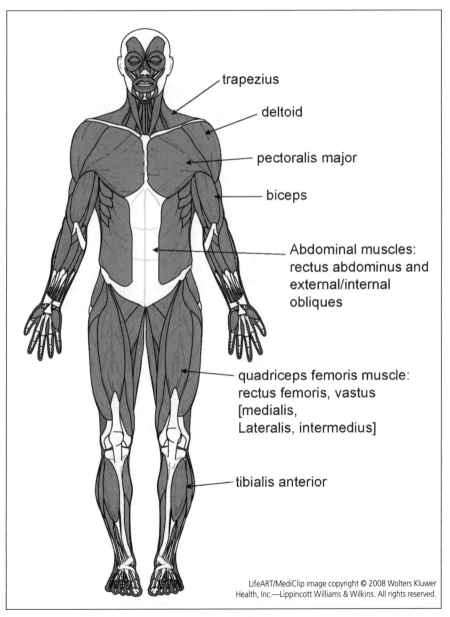

trapezius

deltoid

pectoralis major

biceps

Abdominal muscles: rectus abdominus and external/internal obliques

quadriceps femoris muscle: rectus femoris, vastus [medialis, Lateralis, intermedius]

tibialis anterior

The major muscles, front view.

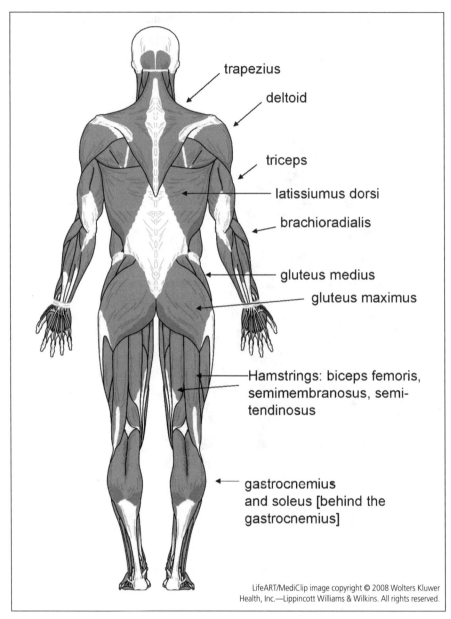

The major muscles, rear view.

- trapezius
- deltoid
- triceps
- latissiumus dorsi
- brachioradialis
- gluteus medius
- gluteus maximus
- Hamstrings: biceps femoris, semimembranosus, semi-tendinosus
- gastrocnemius and soleus [behind the gastrocnemius]

Throwing

Upper Body

Rotator cuff (teres minor, infraspinatus, supraspinatus, and subscapularis muscles). These muscles generate the force to throw and decelerate the arm after throwing the ball. Essentially, the rotator cuff keeps the shoulder stable in a shallow ball-and-socket joint.

Trapezius muscle. Facilitates elevation (upward), depression (downward), abduction (away from the midline of the body), and adduction (toward the midline of the body) movement of the shoulder girdle. It might be the most underrated and neglected shoulder stabilizer.

Forearm pronators. Specifically the pronator teres, which places the hand in a palms-down position. Imbalance or weakness can result in damaging the medial or ulnar collateral ligament, which could necessitate the commonly performed Tommy John surgery.

Forearm supinators. Places the hand in a palms-up position. This also includes the biceps muscle, which acts as the major flexor of the forearm.

Forearm flexors (biceps, brachialis, and brachioradialis). These act as decelerators of the forearm.

Wrist flexors. Facilitate flexion and ulnar deviation.

Deltoids (anterior, lateral, and posterior heads). Aid in acceleration and deceleration of the arm, as well as overall stability of the shoulder joint.

Throwing, Swinging, and Fielding

Trunk

Core (erector spinae, iliopsoas, obliques, and rectus abdominus). These are involved in extension, flexion, lateral flexion (side-to-side), and rotation of the spine. The body is in all positions when fielding. Even though the rotation during a swing is basically level, side-to-side and diagonal strength contributes to the entire swing. Although not all of these muscles are the primary movers for the diagonal twisting motion (throwing), the strength of all the core muscles contributes to diagonal strength.

Lower Body

The lower body provides support and power delivery to the throwing motion. Again, as with the throwing motion, a strong lower body provides support so power can be delivered to the swing. The lower body is also involved in movements in all directions when fielding.

Glutes. The gluteus maximus adducts (moves toward the midline of the body) and extends (moves backwards) the thigh.

Hamstrings (biceps femoris, semitendinosus, semimembranosus, and gracilis). Flexes (moves to the back of the thigh) the lower leg and extends (move backwards) the hip.

Quadriceps (rectus femoris, vastus lateralis, vastus medialis, and vasuts intermedius). These muscles extend (straighten) the lower leg. The rectus femoris also flexes (moving the thigh upward) the hip.

Swinging

Upper Body

Strength in the forearm and grip means a good balance of strength among all the muscles. All the muscles should be properly trained, with no muscle in the area being ignored, although the emphasis would be greater for some muscles than others.

Forearm pronators. Specifically the pronator teres, which places the hand in a palms-down position—for example, the top hand of a batter's grip during the follow-through of the swing.

Forearm supinators. Including the biceps, the supinators place the hand in a palms-up position—for example, the bottom hand of a batter's grip during the follow-through of the swing.

Forearm flexors (biceps, brachialis, and brachioradialis). These muscles lengthen during a swing, but their strength is needed for balance in the forearm and power delivery during the swing.

Wrist flexors. Facilitate flexion and ulnar deviation.

Wrist extensors. Facilitate extension and radial deviation.

Running

You do not need to be the author of a book to know that the trunk and legs are involved in running. However, to know that the lower body and core are involved is not enough information to design a comprehensive program enabling athletes to move fast. Understanding what muscles are involved in locomotion will help when evaluating injury or weaknesses in running technique. The contribution of some muscles to movement is greater than others. For instance, the value of the back of the leg (hamstrings and glutes) far outweighs any attention paid to the quadriceps or trunk. Choosing exercises to properly train the leg for balance will be determined by the muscles involved and their actions during movement.

Trunk

Core. Erector spinae, iliopsoas, obliques, and rectus abdominus are involved in extension, flexion, lateral flexion (side-to-side), and rotation of the spine.

Lower Body

Glutes. The gluteus maximus adducts (moves toward the midline of the body) and extends (moves backwards) the thigh.

Hamstrings (biceps femoris, semitendinosus, semimembranosus, and gracilis). These flex (move to the back of the thigh) the lower leg and extend (move backwards) the hip.

Quadriceps (rectus femoris, vastus lateralis, vastus medialis, and vasuts intermedius). These extend (straighten) the lower leg. The rectus femoris also flexes (moving the thigh upward) the hip.

Note that only the major muscles are listed in these common baseball movements. For example, the lower arm muscles listed in the swing are critical, but the upper arm, chest, and upper back are active as well. However, when speaking of the swing, the forearm plays a more important role, while the other muscles are part of the training for balance and total body strength.

FACT OR FICTION?
BASEBALL TRAINING MYTHS

Before you begin this journey of physical development, it may be helpful to identify some of the training hearsay that has affected baseball since its beginnings. Over the years, training myths and inaccuracies have negatively affected the development of players who wanted to undergo training but felt they would risk injury based on the information they received. Of all today's sports, baseball might be the most impacted by old wives' tales and false premises. These, however, can be easily dispelled by available scientific and evidence-based information. It's a shame that some of these traditional half-truths still persist. Let's take a look at some of the baseball training myths and identify the truths that will enable you to create a fundamentally sound approach.

Myth: Weight training will ruin a good swing and a good arm.

Fact: Nothing could be further from the truth. In fact, weight training can add more power to a swing and produce a healthier, stronger arm! However, if you are planning to lift weights without proper stretching, conditioning, and skill work (fielding, hitting, throwing, and baserunning), then plan to become muscle-bound while ruining your swing and your arm. If you follow the baseball-specific program detailed in this book while practicing your game skills, there is little chance of becoming muscle-bound.

It is the integration of physical training and skill work that helps all athletes get into game-ready shape without decreasing their performance levels. If you expect to properly develop, then the time spent on the baseball diamond should easily eclipse the time spent on physical training. That being said, adding strength will increase the power of a swing. Arm strength and health improves when a pitcher or fielder combines the proper strength program with an appropriate throwing schedule.

Myth: Pitchers should not lift weights.

Fact: If hitters are going to be hitting the weight room, becoming bigger and stronger, then pitchers will have to do the same to keep up. Firsthand experience with Major League pitchers tells us that it is no coincidence that many of the game's premier pitchers are committed to a year-round program. These highly trained athletes are pitching upwards of 200 innings per year, which tells us one thing—they are rarely injured. That is really the key, not only for pitchers but for all baseball athletes: the less injured you are, the more able you are to practice and hone your skills in order to compete at a high level on a daily basis. It is this kind of consistency that leads to career years—and added years to a career.

Myth: Heavy weights tend to make a baseball athlete "tight" and "bulky."

Fact: It's just the opposite—heavy weights make you stronger without producing tightness. First, how do we define "heavy weights?" Is it 100 pounds, 200 pounds, or 500 pounds? What's heavy for one athlete might not be heavy for another. If two people perform the leg press with 500 pounds, one performing twelve repetitions and the other three repetitions, then "heavy" has a different meaning for both. Secondly, a heavy weight should only allow for a few repetitions by definition; one cannot lift a heavy weight numerous times. Competitive weightlifters are a great example of lower repetitions not producing bulk or inflexibility. Classified by body weight, weightlifters train with maximum poundage in the lower repetition ranges, yet maintain their body weights for years while continuing to gain strength. In summary, it appears that lower repetitions performed with heavier weights will produce results that are contradictory to what most baseball people believe.

Myth: For strength and increased flexibility, one should perform workouts with lighter weights and a higher repetition range.

Fact: This is the same thought often held by those who subscribe to the "heavy weight" myth. The problem is that lighter weights and higher repetitions build the least amount of strength and power.

Let's combine the weight gain (bulky and tight), strength, and flexibility issues. Ever checked out a bodybuilding magazine's mass-building (e.g., weight gain) workout? What you will see detailed is higher repetitions (8–15) with lighter-than-maximum weights. Even though the weights are heavier than the normal person can work with, it is not nearly as heavy as it would be if the repetition range was 1–5. Bodybuilders are constantly striving to increase muscle mass. While their physiques are perfectly suited for their sport, they would have flexibility issues when swinging a bat or throwing a ball.

Coaches have supported the use of lighter weights and higher repetitions based on the theory that this type of workout maintains strength, reduces soreness and fatigue, and maintains flexibility. In reality, you will not achieve optimal strength from this type of program, so maintaining strength is out of the question; the reduction of soreness and fatigue is due to the "easiness" of the program; and the stress of the program is so light that it would be nearly impossible to gain weight and lose flexibility. Remember that baseball is a sport that places a premium on speed, power, and agility, and as such you need to "recruit" those muscle fibers that are typically used in the sport.

If you have a program that is too light to keep someone strong and too light to promote muscle growth, why weight train at all? "I am going to lift light weights and get strong" makes little sense and has proven to be the least effective way to gain strength.

Myth "No lifting for me! I know a player who hurt himself while weight lifting. Even after he got over his injury, it seemed as if he always had some nagging problem."

Fact: At times, it can be difficult to determine if someone hurt themselves *because* of weight training or *during* weight training. That is to say, many injuries occur because of a number of factors that have built up over time. There is one thing for certain—weight training has never ruined a career! However, a weight-training program that is improperly supervised and poorly designed will definitely prevent an athlete from progressing to the next level. That is why it is critical that a comprehensive program be designed by a competent, certified strength and conditioning professional so the theories and methods used can be scientifically explained and substantiated by experience and results.

Myth: The forearms are the most important muscles in hitting.

Fact: Although the forearms are no doubt important, gripping strength is an even bigger factor. Without a strong grip (the hands and the fingers), you will never be able to use the forearms efficiently. Did you know that the typical forearm exercises—flexion and extension—are the least common actions used in a swing or a throw? A program uses exercises that maximize grip strength and promote greater strength in the forearms. That being said, hitting for power is a total body product. The body works as a unit, and it should be trained as a whole for the most powerful swing. The exercise menus in this book will be more basic than what most athletes have been exposed to. A total body workout, with specific emphasis on exercises to help the baseball athlete, is the key to maximizing all the necessary physical attributes.

Myth: Weight training in the off-season is fine, but lifting during the season will make you tired and is counterproductive.

Fact: Fatigue is a fact of life in the game of baseball. Simply put, the in-season program is the most important link to the off-season program, and the off-season program is the most important link to the in-season program. Will you be tired if you weight train during the season? If you plan on waiting until you are rested to lift weights, here's a news bulletin: that day will never come. Sure, you will be slightly rested in the beginning if you decide not to lift during the season. However, at the halfway point, you will begin to lose strength, size, and power when you need it the most. An in-season program enables a player to kick it into high gear when the "dog days" of summer beat down those who have done nothing. Weight training is counterproductive only when you are on the wrong program. A year-round training program is the only way to take your game to the highest levels.

Myth: Weight training will make an athlete a better hitter or pitcher.

Fact: Wrong, wrong, wrong! It may seem strange reading this in a book about training for baseball, but weight training alone has never developed good pitchers or hitters and never will. The truth is that if you don't have the components to be a good hitter (e.g., selectivity, good swing, hitting knowledge, vision) or pitcher (e.g., throwing mechanics, knowledge of the hitter's strengths and weaknesses, command of your pitches), then strength will serve no purpose. Being stronger can't help you distinguish a fastball from a change-up or make you throw strikes. However, if you are a good hitter, then development through proper weight training might turn singles into doubles, doubles into home runs, and line drives into moon shots! Increased strength for a pitcher not only results in additional miles per hour on the fastball, but more importantly, a harder slider, a sharper curve ball, a devastating change-up, and a healthier arm.

Myth: "Ruth and Koufax are Hall of Famers, and they didn't weight train, so why should I?"

Fact: Because you are not Ruth or Koufax! For every great athlete who does not train, there are dozens who do. And, as of this writing, since 1936 only 213 of the 260 Hall of Fame members have been voted in as players, so the odds don't look good for you. We know for sure that being in peak physical condition is neither a necessity nor a guarantee for stardom. But it is no coincidence that those committed to a year-round training program have fewer injuries, less severe injuries, outnumber those who don't train, *and* have great years! A good theory to remember is that of the bell-shaped curve. On either ends of the bell-shaped normal distribution (roughly 16 percent per side) are those athletes who might or might not weight train and who might or might not be injured. However, the remaining 68 percent of the athletes in the middle of the curve are healthier, weight train, and have good careers. The middle of the bell-shaped curve is where a well-planned strength and conditioning program can make the most contribution. In the final analysis, the majority of baseball players benefit greatly by a year-round, comprehensive training program.

Myth: An unsuccessful athlete must not have a training program worth looking at.

Fact: This is as irresponsible as believing that a successful athlete *must* have a good program; it is another ignorant statement that will limit the available resources for becoming a great player. There are many variables that go into successful or beneficial programs, and likewise, athletic failure can result from a number of things. Time and again, baseball presents circumstances that are out of the athlete's control. But one thing that can be controlled is the state of physical conditioning. A sound training program will give you all the physical qualities to be a great ballplayer. Using those qualities to your benefit depends on your work ethic on the field.

2

Be the Best Conditioned Ballplayer

Nowhere is the understanding of energy sources, discussed in Chapter 1, more important than when designing a baseball-conditioning program. Years ago, there wasn't much conditioning being done in or out of season. Today, long-distance running or cardiovascular training sessions lasting 20–40 minutes continue to be thought of as a beneficial way to condition the baseball player. *There could not be a worse way to physically prepare for a baseball season.* Sure, today's game looks easy, played in three hours or so, and a fielder might not move much for five innings, but to understand conditioning, today's player needs to grasp basic physiological concepts and maintain an objective, evidenced-based evaluation of what it takes to play the game daily, weekly, and monthly.

THE PROBLEM WITH LOW-INTENSITY CARDIOVASCULAR TRAINING

To be sure, 20–40 minutes of low-intensity cardiovascular training (running, biking, or elliptical trainer) is beneficial for fat loss, body weight maintenance, or improvement in low-intensity endurance. Aerobic exercise is not a waste of time. However, if conditioning should closely mimic game movement and intensity, it is easy to see that low-intensity endurance training has very little to do with preparing an athlete for one game, let alone an entire season.

If you have run continuously for 30 minutes or observed someone doing the same, you would experience these things: 60 to 70 percent effort (estimated); a steady, moderately paced breathing pattern; medium pulse rate (130–156 beats per minute); and fatigued but not "burning" legs. Is this the type of training that prepares a player for a game? Absolutely not! A player "legs out" a double, or an outfielder runs down a ball in the "gap." A pitcher may field a bunt, back-up third base for an overthrow, and cover home after a wild pitch, all in a four-pitch span. While sliding into third base, a runner kicks the ball away from the third baseman, then quickly gets up and sprints home. Low-intensity running does not simulate or prepare the body for these game-like conditions.

Baseball requires 100 percent effort whenever effort is required. As a result of that effort, the athlete will experience high to very-high pulse rates (over 180 beats per minute) and rapid breathing patterns. Teaching the legs to react under these circumstances without breaking down can only be done through high-intensity conditioning that should regularly lead to the "burning" muscle sensation that lower level work cannot accomplish. Frankly, many players with lower body injuries, specifically hamstrings, are injured because they don't condition intensely enough. In other words, they have not trained their bodies to move at top speed or peak effort. So, when it comes time to perform an all-out effort, it is too much of a shock to the body.

THE MOST EFFECTIVE CONDITIONING WORKOUT

Coaches and athletes: take the guesswork out of conditioning. Do not mistakenly use a percentage of effort to determine speed during conditioning workouts. Ballplayers might be asked to run at 50 percent speed or three-quarters speed, but other than track athletes, who knows how fast that is? This type of workout design really amounts to guessing, but guessing does not get the job done. While track and field workouts are based on the percentage of maximum speed over a certain distance, it is nearly impossible to do the same for a ballplayer because there is no given "best time" for the many distances one might run during a game or during training.

Other traditional baseball conditioning programs assign random distances during a running workout without a plan or clear objective. Examples like "run to the gap," "jog to the pole," and "run ten sprints" illustrate a lack of planning. A player wouldn't be asked to guess or esti-mate pitches thrown or number of outs recorded. It makes sense to be as accurate as possible when determining the conditioning effort (speed or intensity) and work (rest intervals and distances covered) so you know the cause and effect.

So, then, what is the most effective design for a conditioning workout? Interval training and jog, stride, sprint! Interval training has little use for continuous distance running, performing a greater amount of work with greater intensity. Jog, stride, and sprint are assigned speeds: jogging is slightly faster than walking; strides are 100 percent effort and approxi-mately 75 percent speed; and sprinting is 100 percent effort and 100 per-cent speed. This allows the baseball athlete to know exactly how fast to run.

INTERVAL TRAINING

Performing a greater amount of work with greater intensity in shorter periods of time builds speed, strength, and endurance. Anyone interested in those qualities? Interval training, which does not have to be restricted to running, is the way to go. The key is maintaining a higher intensity level with short rest periods between runs.

For example, sprinting 400 meters (about a quarter mile) in 70 seconds (average speed of 8.75 seconds per 50 meters) would be a good time for a nontrack athlete. But take that same 400 meters and break it into eight 50-meter segments with a rest period between repetitions, and it can be cov-ered in 56 seconds (7 seconds per 50 meters) or less! Players log faster times over the same distances; with rest intervals, they run farther in a given time than in one continuous run; and finally, they perform a greater amount of work in a given time. In training terms, this is the most effective way to con-dition athletes. This can be done at any distance or for any amount of time.

SPEEDS AND TECHNIQUES
Jog

A jog is technically hard to describe, but you know what it is when you see it. It is the speed just above a walk but below a run; it's warm-up speed. Jogging should never be a training speed but rather a speed that is used while recovering from, or in between, workouts. Or it's the kind of speed used prior to a flexibility and warm-up session.

Strides

A stride is an exaggerated running style at top speed. The normal stride is lengthened as far as possible, yet one must remain conscious not to (a) extend the foot or the lead leg out in front of the body, (b) have an excessive or technically incorrect arm swing, and (c) excessively or intentionally rotate the hips to increase stride length.

The best way to find your stride length is to begin jogging and then slowly lengthen your stride, slightly increasing speed without disrupting correct running technique. When the proper stride length is found, increase speed without shortening the stride but maintaining the new stride length. Again, the effort is 100 percent but the speed is reduced (to approximately 75 percent) because the stride *length* is exaggerated and the stride *rate* (strides per distance or time) is decreased. Additionally, because the stride is lengthened, there is a greater stress (the good kind) on the lower back, glutes, and hamstrings, thus building strength into the run as well as conditioning.

Distances are an important factor, but do not get carried away with longer distances. What you might lack in distance is made up for in higher intensity sprinting. Between 10 and 150 yards (30–450 feet) is more than enough distance considering that the athlete should perform two or more sets of strides.

Aside from sprinting, strides while baserunning are the most specific running drill for baseball. Frankly, there are no better running drills for fielders, because strides provide baserunning practice and conditioning in the same drill. Using the distance/interval equation, baserunning is easy to measure by the 90-foot base paths. Strides can be used for singles, doubles, triples, and homers (covering one base, two bases, etc.). A single would be home to first base, or first base to second base, and so on; a double is home to second base, or first to third, etc. For further specificity, the runner can go from home to first base with an aggressive turn, or from first to third from a hit-and-run start, or from third base to home after tagging up. Add in base coaches giving direction, pitchers as visual clues, or reading the ball off the bat while running and you have the best game-like baserunning drill.

Regular interval timing works effectively when there are only a few athletes participating in the drill. When team running is called for, it is more convenient to line up players at the starting point, and when a runner touches the first assigned base, the next runner begins, continuing the drill nonstop until completion.

If you are looking for a fancy, extensive list of conditioning programs, you won't find it here; it's unnecessary. First of all, there is no magic formula for conditioning, only hard work. Second, it's not that complicated—baserunning, changing speeds, and running technique based on times and distances is the most effective way to get prepared!

Sample Stride Interval Workouts

I. Stride 50 yards ten times (10 x 50 yds), with 15 seconds of rest between each repetition; two minutes of full rest after the set; followed by another ten 50-yard strides (10 x 50 yds), with 15 seconds of rest between each repetition.

II. Stride 100 yards ten times (10 x 100 yds), with 30 seconds of rest between each repetition; two minutes of full rest after the set; followed by ten 50-yard strides (10 x 50 yds), with 15 seconds of rest between each repetition.

III. Stride 60 yards ten times (10 x 60 yds), with 18 seconds of rest between each repetition; two minutes of full rest after the set; followed by ten 30-yard strides (10 x 30 yds), with nine seconds of rest between each repetition; two minutes of full rest after the set; followed by ten 10-yard strides (10 x 10 yds), with 3 seconds of rest between each repetition.

Sprints

No secrets here—run as aggressively and as fast as you can! This is an all-out, winner-take-all effort. The key here is to emphasize effort instead of speed, and sprints will help you understand the difference. In fact, in shorter distances (5–15 yards), technique is not nearly as important as effort, much like running off the mound to field bunts. Sprinting workouts from 5–40 yards are of adequate length.

If you are wondering how sprint workouts of 40 yards or less prepare the athlete for longer distances (home to second base or further), the answer is that the 100 percent effort required during sprint workouts combined with longer-distance stride workouts provide the combination for sprinting longer distances. World-class 100-meter, 200-meter, and 400-meter runners rarely run their event's full distance in training. That is not to say that sprint workouts can't be performed on the base paths. Sprint workouts on the base paths should amount to half the distance of the stride workout. Remember, doubles, triples, and home runs are 60-, 90-, or 120-yard sprints. Simply stated, too many of these full-speed efforts can injure athletes. Just keep in mind how much sprinting is being done *off* the base paths and how much stride work is done *on* the base paths.

We are not necessarily looking for a cardiovascular effect during sprint workouts. We get that from stride running, baserunning, and drilling. To have quality runs during every repetition, it is necessary to have full recovery between each repetition, so athletes should take as much time as necessary between efforts to guarantee repeated top speed. To further ensure quality, the amount of sprinting should be based on distances. Typical sprinting programs have athletes performing 20–30 repetitions at twenty yards or longer. There are two reasons this is not necessary within this conditioning program: there is enough conditioning effect from the stride workout, making it unnecessary for high volume sprinting, and after several long-distance sprints, speed is reduced from fatigue anyway.

Sample Sprint Workouts

To add baseball specificity, begin in a fielding or baserunning stance, or act as if throwing a pitch and preparing to field your position.

    I. 20 x 5 yards (20 sprints @ 5 yards distance)

    II. 12 x 25 yards

    III. 6 x 40 yards

Sample Baserunning Sprint Workouts
(in order of increasing difficulty)

    I. Six times, home to first base; two times, first base to third base; two times, second base to home.

II. Six times, home to first base; three times, first base to third base; two times, first base to home.

III. Six times, home to first base; two times, second base to home; two times, first base to third base; one time, first base to home; one time, home to home.

TIMING

The conditioning effect is directly related to the rest intervals between repetitions and sets. The interval between repetitions determines the majority of the training result, while the rest between sets has more to do with the preparing for the next set. The shorter the break between sprints, the more intense (difficult) the workout will be. A recommended repetition rest interval is 30 seconds of rest per 100-yard repetition. This would mean 15 seconds of rest for a 50-yard run, 18 seconds of rest for a 60-yard run, 21 seconds of rest for a 70-yard run, etc. A two-minute rest period between sets of 10–15 repetitions is a suggested moderate rest period that can be adjusted based on the number of sets, distances covered, and the fitness level of the athlete.

Stride speed can be determined by dividing the recommended rest interval in half. For instance, the speed for a 50-yard stride with 15 seconds rest will be approximately 7–8 seconds. The fitter, faster runners will be 6–7 seconds, and the bigger, slower runners will be 8–9 seconds.

As the athlete becomes more fit, there will be a need to adjust the intervals and distances to achieve the same conditioning effect. Reducing the rest interval between sets by 10–15 seconds will significantly change the routine, as well as reducing the repetition interval by 10-yard increments (that is, assigning the 40-yard rest interval to a 50-yard run). However, do not change the rest intervals and the distances during the same workout, as that might increase the intensity of the workout too much. Also, altering all of the components at once will make it difficult to determine which change caused the results, good or bad.

All interval programs are based on work ratios for the conditioning effect. We recommend beginning at a 2:1 ratio as described (for example, a 12-second rest following a 40-yard, 6-second stride). And, rather than ramping up the intensity by 1:1 training (very intense), slowly progress by reassigning new intervals as previously mentioned.

DRILLS

Agility, coordination, and skill drills can also be used for conditioning. In fact, these types of drills are a necessity not only for conditioning the ballplayer for the game but also for improving on-field skills. The running program utilizes different speeds based on technique, allowing for different distances and conditioning effects. Because the game requires 100 percent effort and 100 percent speed (regardless of technique), "drilling" should mimic that type of intensity. In terms of determining the distances or rest intervals, most of that will come from trial and error.

Agility and coordination drills usually have set distances, with cones or pylons marking the positions and movement directions. Determining intervals for a 10-yard/10-repetition lateral drill (100 yards of total movement) is made simple because the distance covered is easily computed and all that remains is to assign a rest period. For most short-order drills, the effective rest period will be determined by trial and error. After performing the drill several times, the coach can tell if the rest intervals are good enough to get a conditioning response.

Other modes of conditioning, such as stationary bikes, treadmills, or cross-trainers, should be used only during rehabilitation when athletes may have limited mobility, during the early stages of a 12-month conditioning program, or as occasional substitutes to running on the ground. Ground-based training is the most effective way to condition baseball players, simply because that is where they play. It is a priority for no other reason than once you "hit the ground," everything your body has learned from other modes of training is of little use on the field. To say that one can condition effectively by means other than ground-based activity is inaccurate. Likewise, to say that other means of training are similar or identical is false. Alternative training modes are valuable additions for variety, as well as offering cardiovascular benefits. However, the best physical results will come from ground-based training.

INCREASING BASEBALL SPEED

Whoever said you can't improve speed is wrong! Granted, each human has a limited speed potential, but very few athletes ever reach the maximum point. This means that nearly every athlete can improve, especially baseball players. Why? Because baseball speed is not dependent on the straight-ahead speed that other sports are measured by. Baseball speed is seldom straight ahead or over long distances and is not only based on running fast.

Offensive speed is never solely based on a time from home plate to first base; it is a combination of home to first base, base-stealing and base-running knowledge, and skills. Defensive speed is never defined by a 40-yard sprint; it is measured by the ability of infielders to get to the "hole" and outfielders to "run down" fly balls, which has more to do with positioning and reaction time than pure speed. Some improvements in baseball speed don't require any running at all. Along with great conditioning, you can become faster by becoming smarter.

Proper Mechanics

It's true that being a faster runner on the baseball field starts with education. Learning to run correctly is the place to start. If you cannot run correctly, all else is meaningless in terms of gaining, producing, and maintaining speed. Technique does not have to be perfect, nor should technical work take too much time away from hitting, throwing, and fielding drills. Yet there still must be some basic execution of running skills—correct body lean while running, swinging the arms high enough with a good angle at the elbow joint, and lifting the knee high enough for the best stride. The scope of this book is not nearly wide enough to cover running techniques, but there are many other books, tapes, and DVDs by competent speed-improvement coaches—look for a Certified Strength and Conditioning Specialist (CSCS)—that can put you on the right track to improving mechanics.

Reaction Time

Probably the most overlooked and misunderstood quality of baseball speed is reaction time. Reaction time should be considered in every speed-improvement discussion. Coaches talk about a lack of range or speed in a player and suggest strength training or a personal speed coach to solve the problem. In reality, many times the player lacks the ability to "read the ball" off the bat. Above average speed is difficult to see if a runner can't get a good jump when stealing. All these are matters of reaction time.

Reaction time is defined as the time it takes between the running cue and actually running. In a 100-meter sprint, for example, reaction time is the time between the starting gun being fired and the moment the athlete initiates his or her movement out of the blocks. In baseball, it would be

Plyometrics

Entire books have been written on the topic of plyometrics. Plyometrics are based on the theory that the most force a muscle can produce is when it is first stretched (eccentric contraction) and then quickly contracted (concentrically). This *stretch/shortening* cycle is used in skipping, bounding, jumping rope, hopping, handclap push-ups, and some medicine ball throws. The scope of this book excludes a detailed look at plyometrics, but we in no way want to diminish the importance of their inclusion in a comprehensive training program. Development of power in both the upper and lower body can help players run faster in every direction, throw harder, and hit the ball farther.

The most important thing to remember is that certain levels of strength must be achieved before performing and fully benefiting from plyometric work. Without the proper strength levels, the risk of injury increases due to the ballistic nature of plyometric workouts. Generally, plyometrics are not exercises for the beginning athlete. Don't be fooled into thinking that plyometrics, either advanced or basic, are the secret formula for ultimate speed, home run hitting, or 100-mph fastballs. There are no shortcuts or breakthroughs for those types of efforts. Preparing the body properly, patience, and commitment to a good work ethic will eventually make you the best player possible.

Volumes of information exist regarding plyometric training. Thoroughly research the topic and find the program that best fits your situation.

seeing a certain pitcher's motion before attempting to steal a base or a fielder reading the ball off the bat before running to the anticipated area in the outfield.

But improving reaction time is not solely based on movement. For a shortstop, fielding a ball "in the hole" (between third base and shortstop) includes knowing where the pitch is thrown and the hitter's tendencies on certain pitches, as well as watching bat speed at the point of contact. Doing these little things will help you get a bigger "jump" when stealing a base or fielding a ball hit in the "hole."

Baserunning

It's not running the bases that is important, it is baserunning—meaning good baserunning knowledge, technique, and habits. Let's take rounding the bases, for example. How important is it to hit the inside of the base with your foot? Hitting the top of the base could mean a bigger than normal turn, thus running an extra 5–10 feet between the bases. Scoring from first base with the poor technique could mean running an extra 10–20 feet, which might mean the difference between "bang-bang" out and "bang-bang" safe!

Good starts while leading off of a base are important for both quickness and limiting extra running distance. For instance, if the arms aren't moved aggressively enough to completely turn the body toward the next base, then the first steps will not be in the straight line that every runner should be on. Shoulders that are not completely turned toward the base will keep any runner from reaching top speed. Time should be spent with a good baserunning coach so that another pair of eyes can let you know where the problem areas are and help you correct them.

For base runners, "getting a jump" means getting a good "read" on the pitchers wind-up and an idea of what pitch might be thrown. Reaction time here amounts to seeing what you are looking for in the pitcher's motion and running when you see it. How many times have you heard that the fastest runners aren't always the best base stealers? Not all base thieves have above average speed, but all of them have a great understanding of pitchers.

Balls hit to the outfield are easily turned into "extra bases" when a runner knows the arm strength and speed of the outfielders, as well as where they are positioned prior to the ball being hit. So you can see that running speed alone is not the only factor in baseball speed, and sometimes not the most important one. Improvement in reaction time can improve fielding range and baserunning speed without any weight training or conditioning. Time is well spent studying this part of the game as part of a winning approach to baseball.

Speed Endurance

No runner is considered fast, no infielder or outfielder is said to have great range, if they can only do it once! Through proper training (interval stride and sprint training), speed can be produced many times in the course of a game and maintained throughout an entire season. This is also closely connected to work in the weight room, as year-round strength training plays an important role in speed production and maintenance. Forget that nonsense that strength training during the season will slow you down or hurt your arm and your swing. The best players in the world not only train during the season but train hard, have less conditioning-related injuries, and continue to play at high levels all year without a late-season decline.

3

Plan Your
Training Year

The best way to develop your physical qualities is to first determine annual goals and then choose specific times of the year to work on certain qualities to ultimately reach those goals. This is called periodization. From time to time, coaches and athletes depend on the advice of others or merely copy a program used by universities, professional teams, or certain individuals. While most universities and professional teams have certified professionals designing their programs, those programs will be based on a philosophy tailored to the facility being used, the level of athlete, and other programming liabilities, such as time constraints or administrative (e.g., coaches, trainers, doctors) input. In essence, even though a program has been used by a successful team, it might not be suitable or successful for anyone else. This is where the value of periodization comes in. Periodized training, based on individual circumstances and needs instead of mimicry, brings about the best results.

Periodization sounds more advanced than it is. In fact, many coaches and athletes use periodization without knowing it. Designing a plan with separate and different programs at specific times of the year is essentially periodizing that year. Refining the yearly approach by setting short-term goals aimed at a year-end objective is the distinction between good plans and bad ones.

To put it into baseball terms, it is necessary to divide the year into parts. The seasonal schedule determines the other parts of the year. The off-season phase begins the day after the last game, even though the actual training might not begin until several weeks later. The preseason phase begins with the year's first baseball practice and ends with the first game. The in-season phase takes place during the baseball schedule.

SAMPLE BASEBALL PERIODIZATION SCHEDULE

Off-Season: 22 weeks
Preseason: 4–6 weeks
In-Season: 24 weeks

Before any weight lifting or conditioning programs are undertaken, there should be a thorough evaluation of all three phases of the previous year, including injury and rehabilitation status. The effectiveness of the previous program (e.g., gains or losses of strength, speed, power, flexibility, etc.) must be assessed prior to designing the next year's program. Changes should then be made to the program based on actual results from the prior year.

Detailed instructions and illustrations for how to properly perform the weight lifting exercises mentioned in this chapter are presented in Chapter Four. Sample workouts for high school, college, and professional athletes are provided in the Appendices.

OFF-SEASON PHASE

This is the time of year for basic physical development, and specific baseball work should be at its lowest level. Because of this, the athlete is afforded the luxury of training hard, long, and as frequently as necessary without worrying about whether or not it will affect baseball skills. This does not mean that baseball work is completely removed. Part of the year-end evaluation is about your past season's on-field performance and the parts of your game that need improvement. Indeed, continuing light practice sessions 1–3 times per week might be a good idea. Without occasional off-season practice, increasing body weight or strength might cause muscular tightness or a change in swinging or throwing mechanics. However, the fact that there are no games to be played, and the beginning of the season is a long way off, puts the priority on training and not on baseball.

SAMPLE OFF-SEASON TRAINING SCHEDULE		
	A.M.	**P.M.**
Monday	Weight training, 45–60 minutes	Conditioning, 30–45 minutes
Tuesday	Weight training, 45–60 minutes	Batting practice and fielding, 30 minutes; conditioning, 30–45 minutes
Wednesday	Day off	Day off
Thursday	Weight training, 45–60 minutes	Batting practice and fielding, 30 minutes; conditioning, 30–45 minutes
Friday	Weight training, 45–60 minutes	Conditioning, 30–45 minutes

PRESEASON PHASE

Depending on the level of the athlete (e.g., high school, college, professional, etc.), the preseason program will last about 4–6 weeks. During this time, the priority shifts from training to baseball work. The training is continued in an effort to retain the off-season accomplishments, but baseball work takes priority over any physical training. The training is designed around the practice sessions so as not to detract from skill work. If there is a need to work longer on baseball skills, then that time will be taken out of the physical training period. You would rather have baseball tire you for training than the other way around.

A long day on the practice field could lead to a lack of enthusiasm for an hour-long weight-training session. It is unrealistic to expect a quality workout if the session is to last sixty minutes. This does not mean that coaches shouldn't expect a 100 percent effort. However, keep in mind that the athletes will be going as hard as they can, but the output is at about three-quarter capacity due to fatigue. To compensate for these conditions, the coach will have to adjust the workouts to get the most productive scenario. Two ways to accomplish this are to (1) expand the number of training days, which will reduce the daily menu and the training time, and (2) keep the number of repetitions low with shorter-than-normal rest periods in between. The weight should be heavier than at higher repetitions yet lighter than the normal lower repetition load.

SAMPLE PRESEASON TRAINING SCHEDULE			
	PRACTICE SESSION	**WEIGHT TRAINING**	**CONDITIONING**
Monday	2–3 hours	15–30 minutes	15–30 minutes
Tuesday	2–3 hours	None	15–30 minutes
Wednesday	2–3 hours	15–30 minutes	15–30 minutes
Thursday	2–3 hours	None	15–30 minutes
Friday	2–3 hours	15–30 minutes	15–30 minutes

IN-SEASON PHASE

During this time, it's all about winning games—nothing is more important than that. The training is secondary to games and practices. However, overall team health is also important. The biggest benefit from training in the in-season is injury prevention, whereas in the off-season it was strength, speed, and power. While pushing the training envelope during the off-season is the best way to produce gains, the in-season intensity remains high, but exercise selection and weight loads are chosen so that the athlete can always recover from the workout to play at the highest levels.

Here is a comparison of off-season and in-season training loads and volumes, illustrating relatively high intensities but a lower volume in-season:

	OFF-SEASON	**IN-SEASON**
Bench Press	85% x 3 x 5 (3 sets x 5 reps at 85 percent)	85% x 3 x 3 (3 sets x 3 reps at 85 percent)
Squats	90% x 3 x 3–4 (3 sets x 3–4 reps at 90 percent)	90% x 2 x 1 (2 sets x 1 rep at 90 percent)
Clean Pull	80% x 5 x 5 (5 sets x 5 reps at 80 percent)	80% x 5 x 2–3 (5 sets x 2–3 reps at 80 percent)

The training should be scheduled after games or early enough before games to allow for proper nutrition and rest. The exercise menu should be much like the preseason, but the rest between sets can be lengthened to allow for a little heavier weight and more recovery. The in-season menu also takes into account long game-days and the fact that some baseball training occurs immediately after games. The last thing a team or player wants to do following a tough loss or a bad day is eagerly attack an hour-long weight-training program. It makes it easier knowing that following those rough days a 15–20 minute workout is the only thing standing between you and going home!

INTERMEDIATE TO ADVANCED PERIODIZATION MODEL FOR BASEBALL

CORE EXERCISES (SQUATS, DEAD LIFTS, BENCH PRESS, ETC.)		
	OFF-SEASON	PRESEASON	IN-SEASON
Intensity	Low-high	Medium-high	Low-high
	60%–100% 1–12RM	80%–90% 1–5RM	50%–90% 1–5RM
Volume	3–5 sets	3–5 sets	1–3 sets
	1–12 repetitions	1–5 repetitions	1–5 repetitions
	3–60 reps/exercise	3–25 reps/exercise	3–25 reps/exercise

SUPPLEMENTAL EXERCISES (LAT PULL DOWNS, BICEP CURLS, LEG CURLS, ETC.)		
	OFF-SEASON	PRESEASON	IN-SEASON
Intensity	Low-high	Medium-high	Medium-high
	5–12 RM	5–8 RM	4–8 RM
Volume	3–5 sets	3–5 sets	1–4 sets
	5–12 repetitions	5–8 repetitions	4–8 repetitions
	15–60 reps/exercise	15–40 reps/exercise	4–32 reps/exercise

Note: Since high school training is primarily developmental and somewhat linear (continual improvement), the periodization scheme shown here illustrates a model primarily for college and professional ballplayers.

RM = repetition maximum. This is the maximum poundage that one can lift in an exercise for a given number of repetitions. For example, 60%–100% 1–12RM (60 to 100 percent of a 1–12 repetition maximum) translates into the maximum poundage you can lift for between one and twelve repetitions. For a 200-pound, one-repetition maximum dead lift, a 60 percent 1RM is 120 pounds. If a maximum of twelve repetitions is performed at 100 pounds in a leg curl, then 100 percent 12RM is 100 pounds.

4

Weight Training Exercises for the Ultimate Baseball Athlete

core exercise group should be established from which all individualized programs are designed. This basic menu of exercises can be used as a definitive structure throughout your training life. The core is a menu that must be efficiently performed before any progressive modifications, additions, or deletions can be made. The following list forms this base menu but is not restrictive when modifications need to be made for injuries or limitations. This is followed by supplemental exercises to complete your baseball workout.

CORE EXERCISES

Bench Press

Chest pressing is an important exercise for most athletes. This type of movement involves a major muscle mass (pectoralis), as well as the shoulders, triceps, and shoulder girdle stabilizers. The preferred chest press is the bench press, where the heaviest weight can be lifted using the most musculature. It might very well be the most effective pressing strength exercise for the upper body. However, sometimes the shoulders or elbow joints are more comfortable pressing at an angle or using dumbbells. So, also listed are some viable alternatives for the bench press if modifications need to be made.

Bench Press

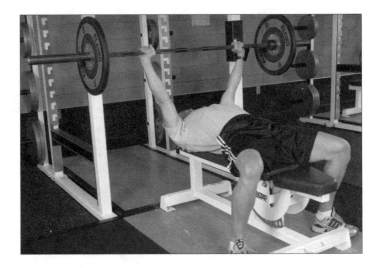

Before taking the starting position, the grip must be determined by the "90-degree rule"—the grip should be such that, at the midpoint of the exercise, the elbow joint should be approximately 90 degrees for the best pressing leverage. Find the grip placement, place the feet firmly on the ground, and remove the bar from the rack, balanced at arm's length.

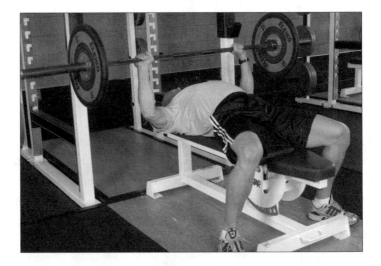

At the midway point, the elbows should be around 90 degrees while slowly but deliberately lowering the bar.

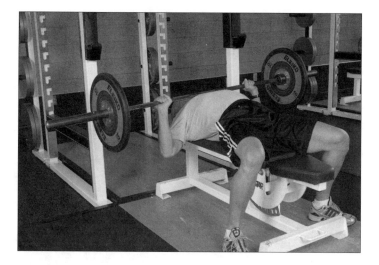

The bar should touch about the midchest region, without pause, before pressing to the starting position.

Comments and Tips

- Don't move the feet. The best bench pressers "push" into their legs without moving their feet at all. Also, moving the feet causes the lifter to lose balance.

- Do not raise the glutes off the bench. "Arching" changes the emphasis on the chest and results in the least amount of development.

- Do not quickly lower the bar and try to "bounce" it off the chest. Bouncing, like arching, results in the least amount of strength and chest development.

- Neglecting the importance of this exercise in a well-rounded program might lead to more upper body injury.

Flat Dumbbell Bench Press

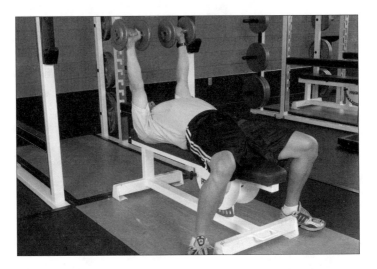

Begin with the hands at arm's length, directly above the shoulders.

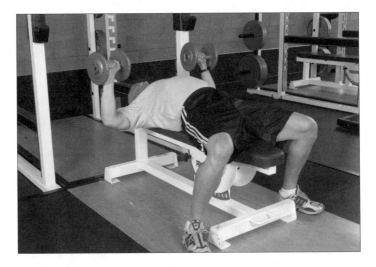

The midpoint is at the same 90-degree angle found in the barbell bench press.

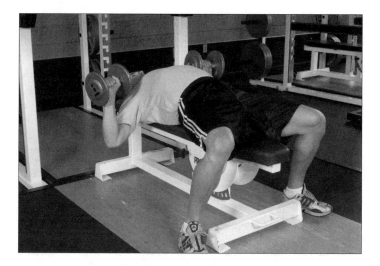

The hands will be closer to the shoulders than with the barbell bench press.

Comments and Tips

- Even though the dumbbells might be close to the body at the bottom part of the lift, they will follow the same path (wide at the midpoint) as when lowering.

- Sometimes the shoulder is uncomfortable with the typical motion and technique. Because of this, it is okay to have the elbows closer to the body than illustrated, and the palms can face inwards.

- Dumbbells are an excellent substitution for a bar if there is a history of shoulder, chest, or arm limitations. Dumbbells allow you to freely move the arms in a motion that better accommodates different body types and upper body structures.

Incline Barbell Bench Press

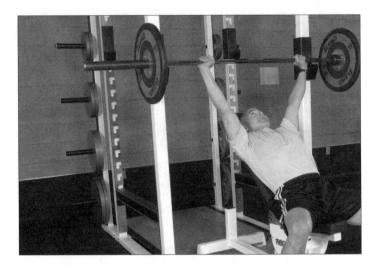

Take the identical grip as in the bench press, unless a wider or narrower grip is easier on the shoulder while pressing. The bench should be positioned at approximately a 45-degree angle.

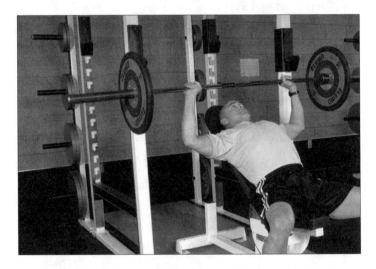

At the midpoint, notice the 90-degree angle at the elbow, which is similar to the flat bench press.

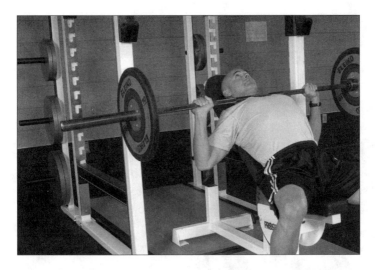

The bar should be brought to touch the body, somewhere between the clavicle (collar bone) and the upper chest. After touching the chest, without pausing, press the bar to the starting position.

Comments and Tips

- As in the flat bench press, keep the feet planted firmly for balance and strength.

- Keep seated during the entire movement; don't raise the hips.

Incline Dumbbell Bench Press

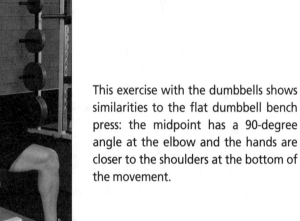

This exercise with the dumbbells shows similarities to the flat dumbbell bench press: the midpoint has a 90-degree angle at the elbow and the hands are closer to the shoulders at the bottom of the movement.

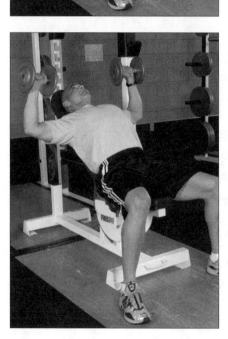

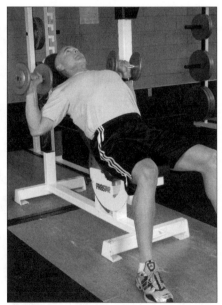

Squats

The squat is the best overall lower body strength exercise and an under-rated, overlooked developer of core (abdominal and lower back) strength. Supervised and performed correctly, this exercise can be the key to strength, increases in muscular size, and increases in speed. At the least, the athlete is asked to balance the body using the ground as the surface—just like in baseball. The back squat appears to be the most effective squatting movement that works the lower back, glutes, and quadriceps. The one-leg squat allows the same lower body flexibility while lessening the load on the lower back for those with lower back issues.

Back Squat

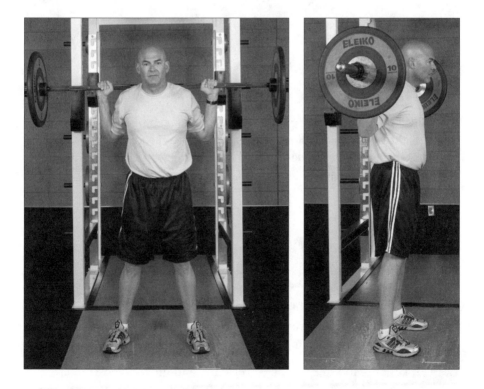

Although the stance should be comfortable and allow for good flexibility, the stance is usually shoulder-width or wider and the bar rests on top of the trapezius.

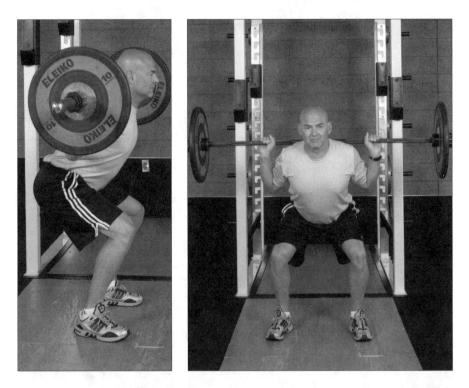

The midpoint or quarter-squat position—begin the squat by keeping the heels flat, back straight, and shoulder blades squeezed together. Bending at the waist, the motion of the hips would be described as "back and down" with very little movement forward at the knees.

Comments and Tips

- The head position should be in line with the back angle throughout the entire movement. "Throwing" the head back when rising out of the squat may leave the lifter unbalanced.

- A squat is too deep if the lower back and glutes "tuck under" the body (rounding of the lower back). This would mean that the first movement when rising is from the lower back, which in time might lead to injury.

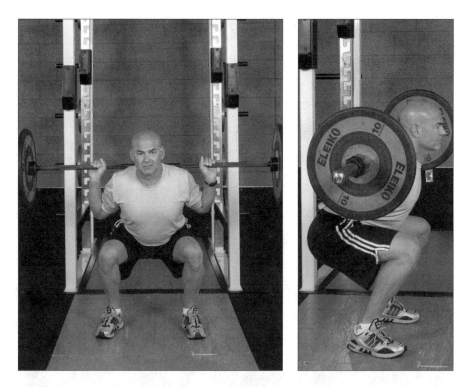

There are varying opinions on the proper depth at the bottom phase of the squat: top of the thigh parallel, bottom of the thigh parallel, or bend of the waist parallel to the top of the knee. The front view shows the important position of the knees in line with the feet. Look at the wall socket in the side views and notice that the position of the knees has changed little, illustrating balance and the "back and down" technique.

- The knees moving inward toward each other at any time during the squat indicates a weakness in the upper leg or lack of flexibility. The squat should be postponed until the technique can be corrected or strength acquired.

- The hips and the shoulders should be rising simultaneously when finishing the lift. If not, it is likely the weight is too heavy or the lifter's back lacks strength.

- As good as this exercise is for the lower body, the squat might arguably be the best exercise for the *entire* body.

One-Leg Squat

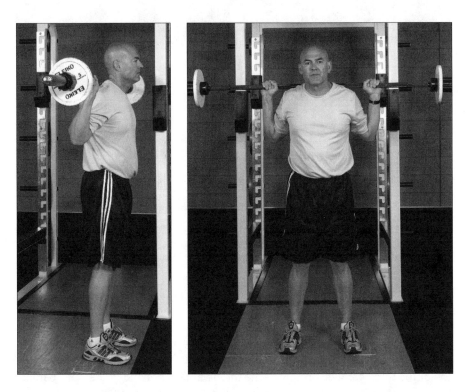

The bar is placed on the upper shoulders and the feet are at, or slightly wider than, hip-width apart.

Comments and Tips

- The upper body should not be entirely upright when lowering or raising the body. Bend at the waist (as in the squat) to effectively train the glutes and hamstrings.

- Do not let the knee on the back leg touch the ground.

- Alternate both legs as opposed to performing all the repetitions on one leg.

- When it comes down to it, single-leg strength is the objective in a training program.

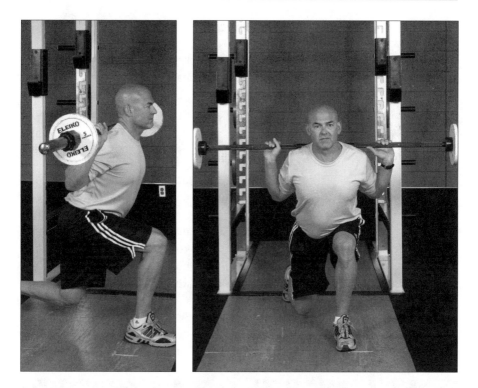

Keeping a straight back, and body weight balanced on the right leg, step back with the left leg while bending at the waist and lower the body until the right knee joint is at roughly 90 degrees. Similar to a squat, as soon as the body reaches the proper depth, immediately rise (do not pause) to the starting position. Correct technique finds the body weight balanced on the "lead" leg throughout the entire movement. Repeat with the other leg.

Olympic-Style Movements from the Ground

Creating basic strength in the lower body by lifting weight from the ground does not sound that exciting, but it remains one of the simplest ways to gain high levels of strength and power. In the case of the baseball athlete, the training of the lower back, hamstrings, and quadriceps has obvious benefits, such as increasing running speed or contributing miles-per-hour to a fastball or bat head speed. The clean dead lift is the primary movement that may or may not progress to the more powerful clean pull. Either way, an Olympic-style movement from the ground is a must for any player if they want to be more powerful.

Clean Dead Lift

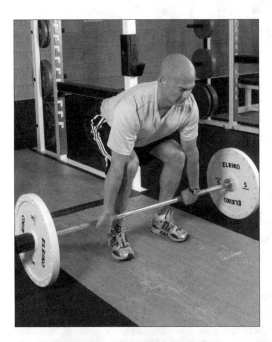

Keep the bar close to the shins, back straight (slightly arched, if possible), shoulders over the bar, arms straight, and elbows rotated outwards.

Lift the bar to the "hang" position using the legs, not the back, and raising the hips and shoulders simultaneously while maintaining a straight back and keeping the bar close to the body. Do not straighten the legs until the lift is complete.

Achieve the upright position by moving the hips to the bar while straightening the legs.

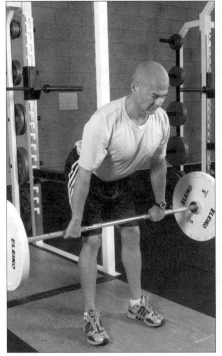
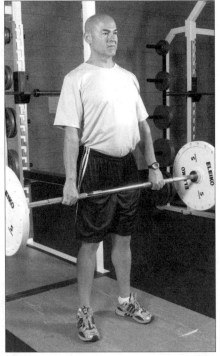

Comments and Tips

- Lifting the bar too fast will result in the legs straightening and all the stress being focused on the lower back. This is the type of technique that will cause lasting back pain. Assuring the correct technique might be determined by using the proper weight.

Clean Pulls

The power clean is a popular exercise for power development in the lower body. However, there is an injury risk to the wrists and hands when performing the power clean. In baseball, you're always catching, throwing, fielding, or swinging with one or both hands, so the small amount of risk is not worth it. Also, the majority of the benefits from this exercise come from the pulling motion as opposed to "cleaning the bar," so why take the risk? A combination of the low back, glutes, and quadriceps producing explosive movement is one of the most sport-specific exercises for a baseball athlete.

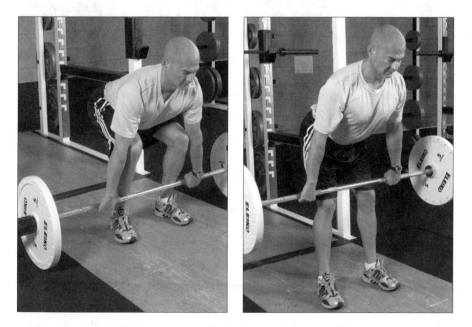

The "jump/shrug" and "pull" phases of the lift are separate moments but are quickly and explosively combined. It is important to separately illustrate the proper techniques. From the "hang" position, there must be an aggressive vertical action that is best accomplished by moving the hips toward the bar, rising up on the toes, and shrugging the shoulders as the arms remain straight.

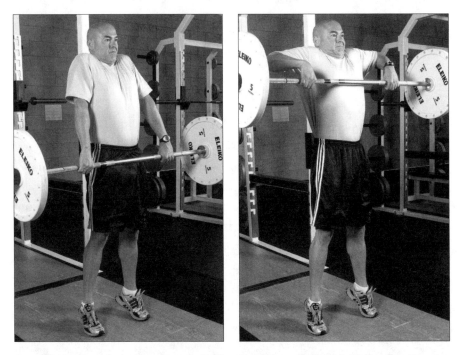

Continue the vertical movement, bringing the bar to chest height by elevating the elbows; "drive" the elbows upward, achieving full body extension with the bar continuing to remain close to the body.

SUPPLEMENTAL EXERCISES

Hamstring Training

The hamstrings are two-jointed muscles (they cross the knee and hip joint) that must be trained with more than one exercise in order to effectively strengthen this area, which balances the dominating strength of the quadriceps. Don't be fooled by a "one hamstring exercise" philosophy. Aggressively training the lower leg flexion is critical for running speed and hamstring health.

Lying Leg Curls

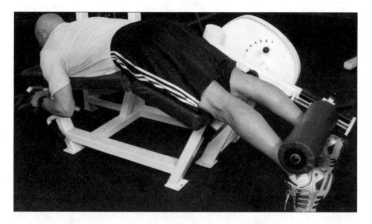

This is the starting position for both one- and two-leg curls.

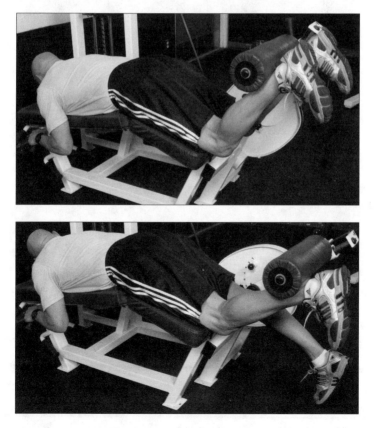

The legs should be in this position at the midway point.

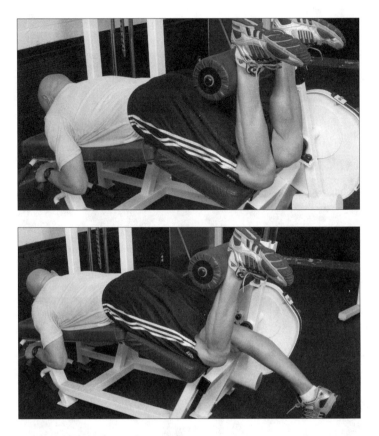

At the finish, keep the hips down.

Comments and Tips

- Do not quickly jerk the lever arm into motion—apply steady pressure with your leg(s).

- The hips should maintain contact with the bench throughout the movement. If this becomes too difficult, then the resistance is too heavy.

- One-leg curls are particularly good for those with back issues or those recovering from hamstring injuries.

- Most athletes and coaches will train the front of the leg more aggressively and consistently than the hamstring complex. This leads to the debilitating hamstring tear because of muscular imbalance or lack of conditioning.

Bent-Leg Dead Lifts

Lower back, glutes, and hamstrings work as a unit when sprinting, throwing, and hitting, so it makes sense to have at least one exercise that works all three in unison. This exercise allows for a heavy weight to be lifted while stressing the backside, which prepares you for dynamic movements on the baseball diamond. Unlike other exercises, the preference for this movement may be decided by flexibility, strength, limitation, and body type. Both of the listed exercises are excellent.

Bent-Leg Dead Lift with Barbell

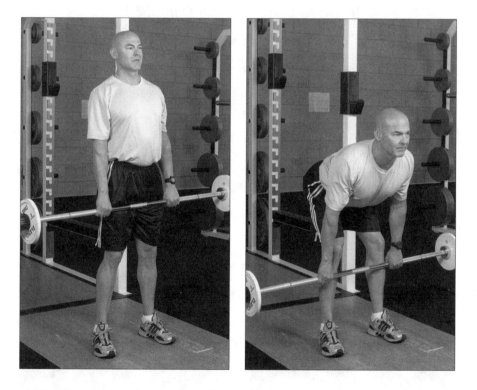

The best way to do this is to push the hips back while bending forward. The feet should be flat, but the body weight should be distributed to the heels. When the bar reaches midshin, return to the starting position.

Comments and Tips

- The slight bend in the knees should not change throughout the entire movement.

- The back must remain straight and flexed, never rounded or relaxed.

- This exercise has also been called an RDL (Romanian dead lift).

Bent-Leg Dead Lift with Dumbbells

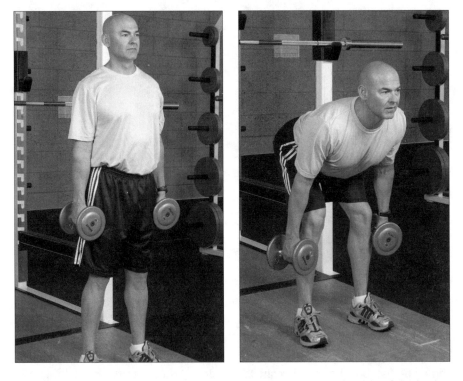

The dead lift with dumbbells allows the weight to remain on the side of the body throughout the entire movement.

Rowing

Rowing involves the largest upper body muscle (latissimus) and several other muscles (rhomboids, trapezius) involved in shoulder and scapular stabilization, as well as the biceps muscles. Rowing is the perfect complementary balance to the bench press. Two-arm rowing allows for the most weight to be handled, but one-arm rowing includes a slight torso rotation, which has a beneficial training effect on left and right twisting movements.

Seated Cable Rows

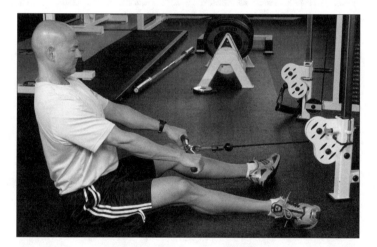

Keep the back straight and legs slightly bent (reducing back stress) while reaching as far forward as possible. There is no reason to lean forward as in a toe-touching position.

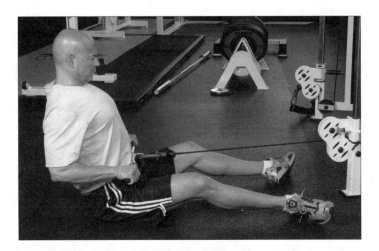

With the chest out and back tight, pull the bar to waist level, concentrating on the "lats" and not the arms.

Comments and Tips

- It is difficult not to use the lower back when using a training weight. The key is to concentrate on the "lats" and not use the back to gain momentum while pulling.

- If the focus is on "driving" the elbows back, then the use of the arms and flexing of the wrist is limited, making the exercise more effective.

One-Arm Cable Rows

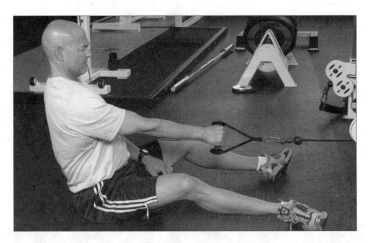

Much like the two-arm row, keep the back straight and reach as far forward as possible, without leaning too far forward or turning the shoulder.

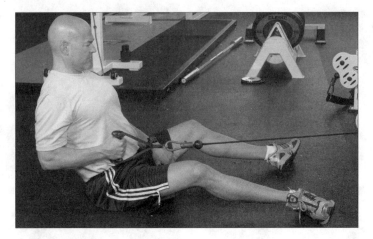

Pull the cable to the hip.

Comments and Tips

- When throwing a baseball, the arm finishes in a full stretched position. Be sure to reach as far as possible at the beginning of each repetition to simulate the stretch at the end of the throwing motion.

- Use an adequate weight to keep the upper body from moving and twisting during the exercise. Limit excessive movement so that the work is done by the "lats" and not the lower back.

Dumbbell Rows

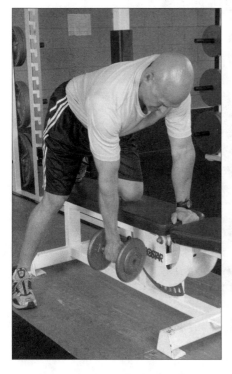 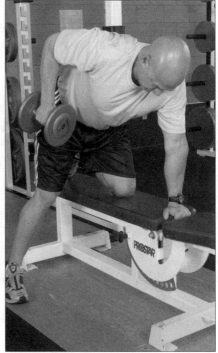

At the beginning of the movement, the back is straight, with one arm holding the dumbbell in a fully stretched position (using the opposite knee on the bench for support) and the other arm bracing the body on the bench.

Pull the dumbbell to the hip.

Comments and Tips

- Pulling the dumbbell to the chest puts more stress on the biceps and less on the latissimus dorsi.

- Be sure to get a full stretch at the bottom of the exercise to simulate the full stretch that occurs in the arm during the throwing motion.

Lat Pull Down

The "lats" need to be stressed from a variety of angles for proper development. Overhead pulling is helpful for strength and flexibility around the shoulder joint. However, be careful not to take a grip with your hands closer than shoulder width apart, as it will put the throwing shoulder in an unfamiliar, stressful position. As a complement to the incline press, the lat pull down is (a) necessary to help balance the front and back of the shoulder and (b) similar to the working angles of the incline press to make the complement perfect. The two-arm lat pull down is the basic strength movement that, depending on progress or individual needs, can be modified to the one-arm lat pull down, which will have a slight torso rotation.

Two-Arm Lat Pull Down

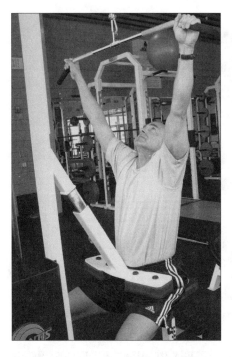 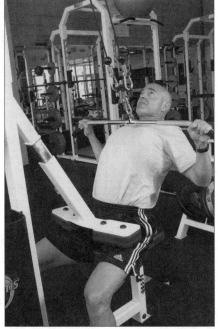

Take a grip that is wider than shoulder-width apart, never a narrower grip. Too wide a grip puts too much stress on the arms. When seated, the bar should be slightly in front of the body.

To begin pulling the bar to the upper chest/collar bone area, lean back slightly but do not use excessive body motion to help pull the bar. Pull the bar straight to the upper chest/collar bone area.

Comments and Tips

- Concentrate on pulling with the elbows for the correct bar path. Pulling with the hands will sometimes bring the bar too low on the body and put more stress on the arms.

- It is important to remember not to use excessive body motion while pulling the bar. It will fool you into thinking you are becoming stronger and could also cause injury.

- The moderate grip evenly stresses the "lats" and arms yet does not put the shoulder in an uncomfortable or compromising position.

One-Arm Lat Pull Down

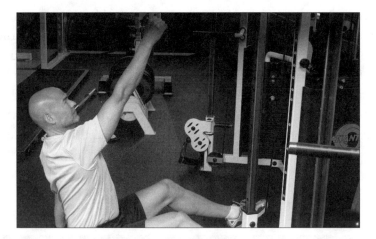

Sit close enough to fully extend the shoulder without having to turn the body to reach the cable. However, if the cable is above your head, you are too close.

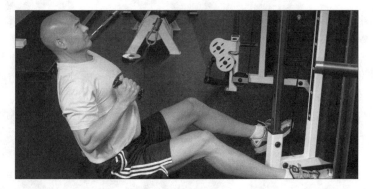

Lean back slightly and pull the cable to the chest. If you pull the cable too low, the "lats" receive little work. Pull it too high and the arms are used more than they should be.

Comments and Tips

- Turning the body while pulling should be kept to a minimum. The chest should be out and the back tight with the concentration on the "lats."

Lateral Shoulder Raise

Anterior and posterior deltoid muscles are affected by most pressing and pulling exercises. The lateral deltoid is one-third of the deltoid structure and is usually ignored in most exercise routines, but it must be directly trained for complete throwing-shoulder health. While the two-arm lateral raises can teach the fundamental motion while building a strength base, one-arm raises will allow you to concentrate on technique and isolation of one deltoid and to use a heavier weight in the advanced stages of training.

Two-Arm Dumbbell Lateral Raise

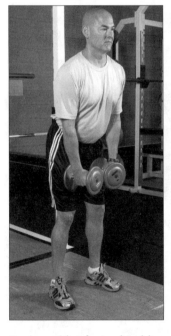 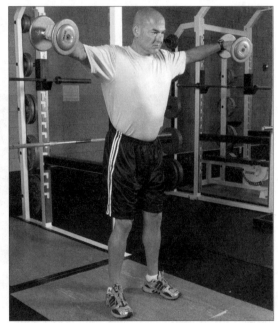

Begin with feet shoulder-width apart, knees slightly bent, and palms facing each other. There should be a slight lean forward.

Raise the dumbbells to shoulder height while maintaining a palms-down position.

Comments and Tips

- Focus on raising the elbows instead of raising the dumbbells. Usually, if the focus is on the dumbbells, the dumbbell ends up higher than the elbows, which lessens the effect on the shoulders.

- Keep the knees slightly bent during this movement.

One-Arm Dumbbell Lateral Raise

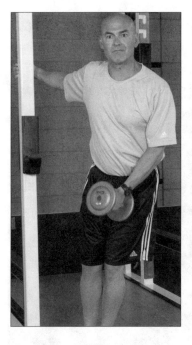 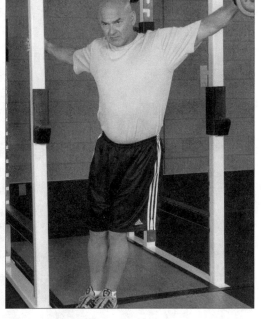

The stance should be such that a straight arm holds the body at an angle; the dumbbell is held at the thigh with a bent-arm position.

Maintain the bent-arm position and raise the dumbbell just above shoulder height. Palms should be facing downward during the lifting part of the movement; maintain the dumbbell parallel to the ground.

Comments and Tips

- It is difficult to keep the dumbbell from rotating upward (thumbs up) when the exercise becomes hard. This should be the factor that decides whether a weight is too heavy or too light.

- The arm that is supporting (holding) the body must be kept straight throughout the exercise.

- The feet should be closer to the support than the shoulders before beginning the exercise.

Rear Deltoid Raise

Weak decelerator muscles can injure both the front and back of the shoulder, as well as the rotator cuff. The posterior deltoid muscle is an impor-

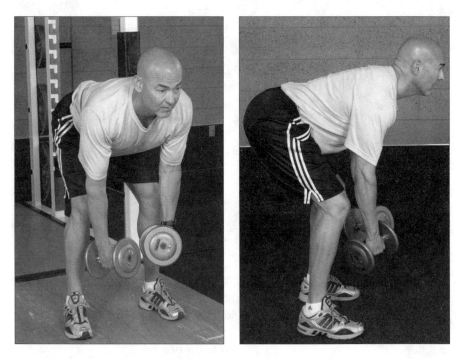

For this exercise, the back should be straight and near parallel to the ground, knees bent, and shoulders *not* rounded.

tant, strong decelerator during the throwing motion. If you want your shoulder to be healthy, there is one muscle you need to include in your training—the rear deltoid. After developing good strength and technique with the two-arm bent lateral raise, one-armed movements might be the next step for improved concentration and further progress.

Two-Arm Bent Lateral Raise

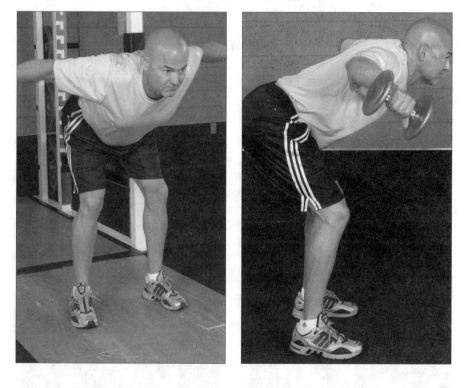

With the elbows slightly bent (which should not change throughout the entire movement), begin raising the dumbbells to the side, keeping the palms facing the ground. Follow the same path while returning the dumbbells to the starting position. The back position should change very little while performing the exercise.

Comments and Tips

- When the thumbs begin to move vertically, the emphasis on the muscle changes and so does the exercise. If anything, point the thumbs toward the ground.

- It is not the height of the dumbbell that matters but rather a full range of motion at the shoulder. Some athletes can raise the dumbbell higher than others.

- Think about raising the elbows instead of raising the dumbbell.

One-Arm Bent Lateral Raise

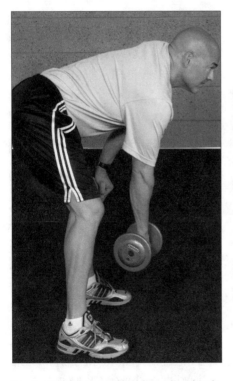 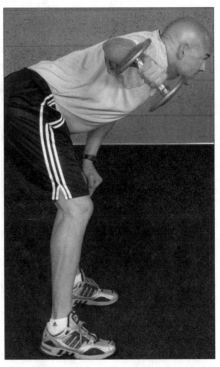

Begin with one arm holding the dumbbell, with the shoulder fully stretched and the opposite arm braced against the knee.

The elbow is slightly bent while raising the dumbbell outward from the body. The elbow angle does not change during the movement, and the shoulders do not turn helping to lift the weight.

Comments and Tips

- Lifting the dumbbell at an angle (the thumb pointing slightly downward) helps to maintain the arm, elbow, and hand position, making for a better exercise.

- Raising the dumbbell close to the body puts more stress on the latissimus dorsi and less on the rear deltoid muscle. The elbow should be away from the body during the exercise.

One-Arm Bent Lateral Raise with Cable

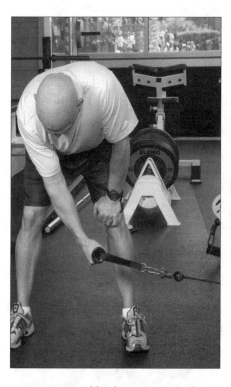

Use an arm and body position similar to the bent lateral raise with the dumbbell, but make sure the hand/cable position starts in front of the opposite shoulder.

Finish the movement at shoulder height.

Comments and Tips

- Finishing the exercise higher than the shoulder line lessens the resistance from the muscle when using a cable.

- The fact that there are three examples of rear deltoid training should be indicative of how important that area is to a healthy, strong arm.

Shrugs

Commonly overlooked, the trapezius muscle is an important scapular stabilizer. Not only does the trapezius raise and lower the shoulder girdle, but it also contributes to forward and backward movement—obviously important to throwing a baseball. Barbell shrugs are effective, but because the bar is held in front of the body and the muscle is behind, they are less than ideal. Dumbbells held at the side of the body put the weight in a better position to affect the "traps" and increase range of motion.

Dumbbell Shrug

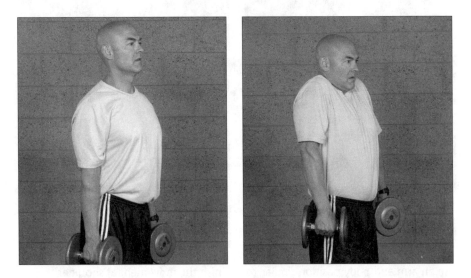

Palms should be facing the body, the arms are straight, and the back (upper and lower) is stiff. The shoulders are not rounded. Bending the legs slightly will reduce any unnecessary tension in the lower back. Shrug (elevate) the shoulders as high as possible while keeping the arms straight.

Comments and Tips

- Rolling the shoulders forward or backward after the shrugging motion adds no significant benefit.

- Use of the legs to "jump" the weight into a shrug will result in less progress.

- Athletes with a history of back injury or those with current limitations can benefit by one-armed shrugs with a dumbbell or by using a cable system. The technique is the same with one arm as it is with two.

Biceps Curls

A ballplayer rarely flexes his biceps muscles in game situations, but training the biceps makes for stronger pulling efforts and stronger decelerators, a healthier arm, and improved upper body balance. Plus, if you're going to train the triceps muscles, you must also train the biceps.

Alternate Dumbbell Curls

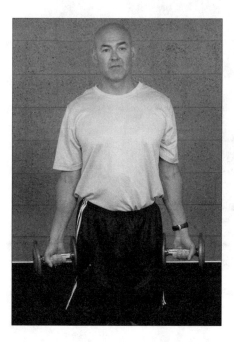

Begin with the dumbbells held with palms facing the body or forward.

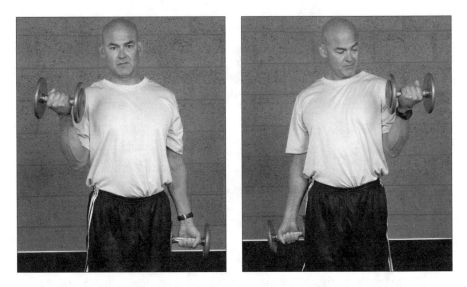

Raise one dumbbell while slightly turning the hand (thumb away from the body), until the dumbbell is at shoulder height. Lower and repeat with the other arm.

Barbell Curls

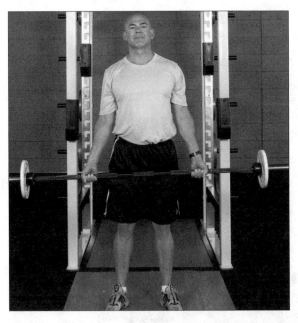

The barbell should be held with a grip slightly wider than the hips.

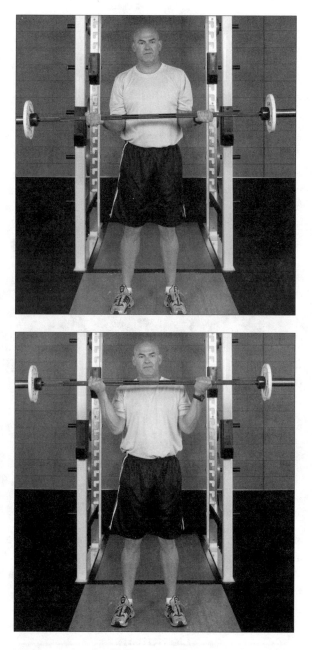

Without using the back or shoulders, raise the barbell to shoulder height, then lower and repeat.

Triceps Extension

If you're going to train the biceps, you must also train the triceps! Similar to the biceps, stronger triceps makes for stronger pushing movements, thus increasing overall strength and balance.

Triceps Push Down

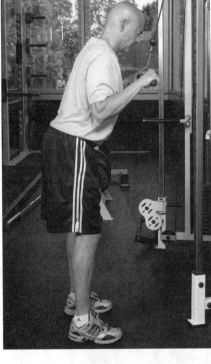 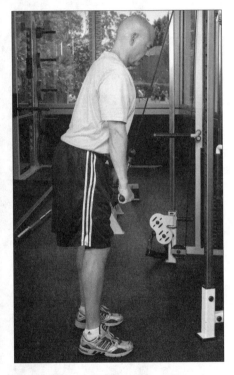

Begin the exercise with the back straight, slightly bent at the waist, and with the legs bent. The elbows should be held close to the body.

Without using the shoulders or chest, extend the arms while keeping the elbows close to the body, until the arms are straight.

Deviation

As the most functional forearm exercise for baseball players, this wrist movement is more useful than the traditional wrist curl (flexion) and reverse wrist curl (extension).

Hammer (Radial Deviation)

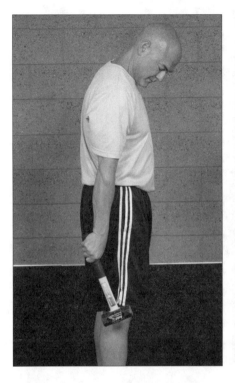 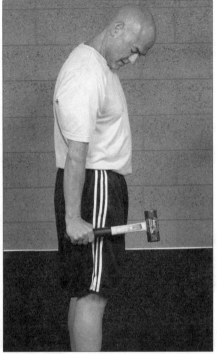

Before the exercise begins, grip the handle while the hammer is perpendicular to the ground. Then put the arm straight to the side while maintaining a tight grip.

Keeping the arms straight, and without the use of muscles other than the forearm, bring the weighted end to the forearm as far as possible.

Comments and Tips

- For the best results, never loosen the grip or bend the arm while performing the movement.

Hammer (Ulnar Deviation)

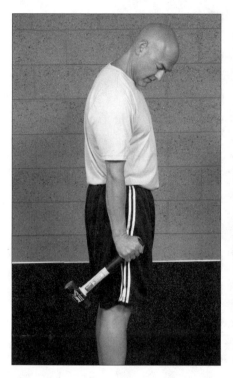 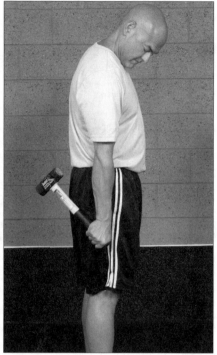

Before the exercise begins, grip the handle while the hammer is perpendicular to the ground. Then put the arm straight to the side while maintaining a tight grip.

Keeping the arms straight, and without the use of muscles other than the forearm, bring the weighted end to the forearm as far as possible.

Grip Strengthening

Strong forearms do not necessarily mean a strong grip. Without a strong grip (fingers and hand), forearm strength cannot be efficiently used. Grip strength should be a key focus for younger players, especially hitters. Using different-sized objects to squeeze is critical to building good gripping strength.

Gripper

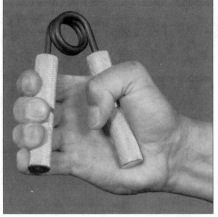 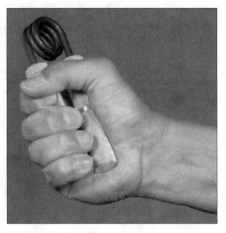

This is typical of a grip-strengthening device. The hand must be in a secure position on the handles in order to perform the exercise.

Squeeze the handles until they touch.

Comments and Tips

- There are varying degrees of resistance amongst grippers. The handles should touch with each repetition for the best result.

Ball Squeeze

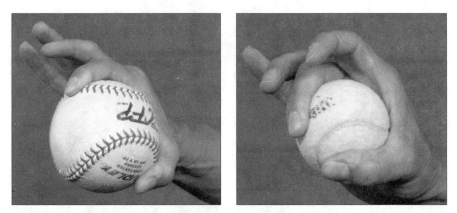

Take the softball or tennis ball and squeeze with every finger.

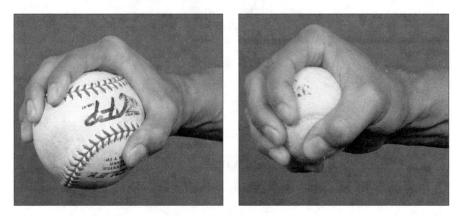

After each single-finger squeeze has been performed, a full-handed squeeze is the final grip to complete one repetition.

Comments and Tips

- A 100 percent effort is necessary for the given amount of time prescribed for squeezing. Don't shortchange one of the most important exercises for hitting-grip strength.

- Using one or two different-sized spherical objects of varying rigidity (soft like a tennis ball; hard like a softball) about every eight weeks is optimal for developing grip strength.

Rotational Abdominal Exercises

Rotation of the trunk is the most dominant baseball movement, and the trunk should be trained for and strengthened. You wouldn't use the same weight on the bench press every workout and expect to get strong! Like any other muscle, the abdominal region must be strengthened by the use of weights, weighted objects, or resistance of some kind (progressive resistance). Several exercises, standing and seated, provide a strengthening effect to the abdominals that will transfer to your swinging and throwing motion. Regular sit-ups and leg raises won't cut it.

Seated Twists

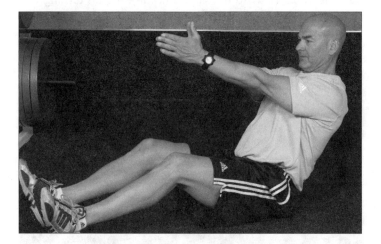

Lean back at about a 45-degree angle (in this example, the feet are unsecured, but they can also be secured under a bench or held by a partner), with arms straight and perpendicular to the body.

Comments and Tips

- Keep the arms locked in place while rotating the body. Often, the arms move more than the upper body.

- Adding weight in this exercise is the *only* way (as for all abdominal

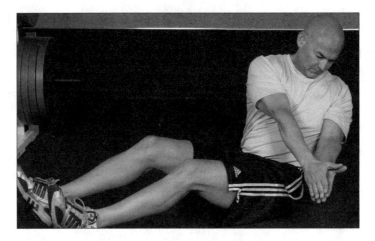

Turn the upper body to the side, concentrating on turning the shoulders while maintaining the arm position.

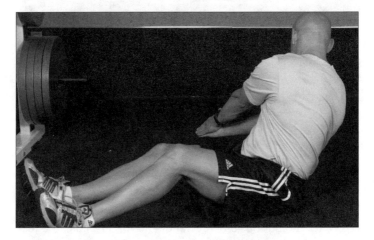

As soon as the shoulders can no longer turn, immediately rotate to the other side and repeat in a continuous, nonstop motion until the prescribed number of repetitions is performed.

exercises) to truly continue to build strength in this region. The weight is held in the same arm position as illustrated.

- Don't expect continual strength gains when working the abdominals if there is not resistance added.

Lying Twists

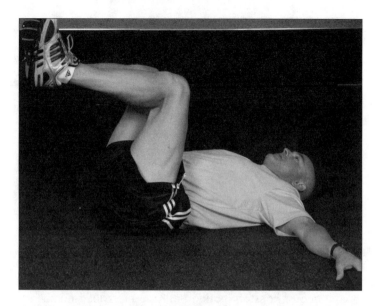

Begin lying on the back, arms perpendicular to the body, palms down, and feet off the ground, knees bent at 90 degrees.

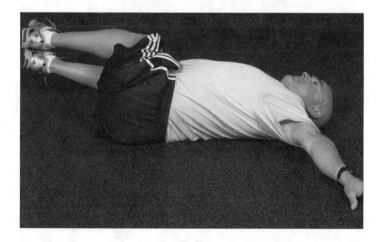

Maintain the upper body position and rotate the lower body to one side, while also maintaining the position of the legs and feet. The body should rotate at the midback (thoracic) position.

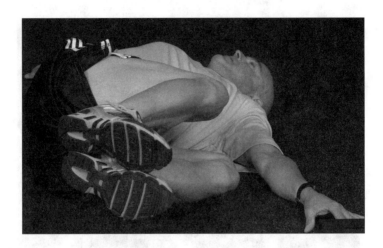

After fully rotating (the legs should touch but not rest on the ground), immediately rotate in the other direction and repeat in a continuous, nonstop motion until the prescribed number of repetitions is performed.

Comments and Tips

- Although the arms are used to secure the upper body position, concentrate on rotating the body at the trunk instead of "pushing" the ground with the palms.

- Never relax the abdominals during the movement. Changing directions while rotating with relaxed abdominals might round the back and, over time, cause injury or unnecessary soreness.

Standing Twists

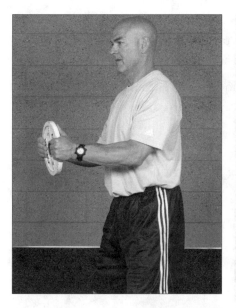 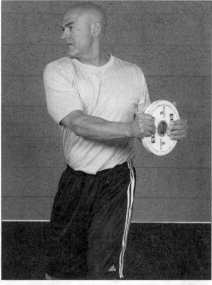

Stand with your legs slightly bent and the elbows fixed at 90 degrees, with the upper arms close to the body.

Twist to one side, moving the arms and shoulders together. The head should be focused forward, and the objective is to move with the opposite side shoulder to the chin.

As soon as the shoulder and chin meet, repeat to the other side and continue, alternating to each side nonstop for the prescribed number of repetitions.

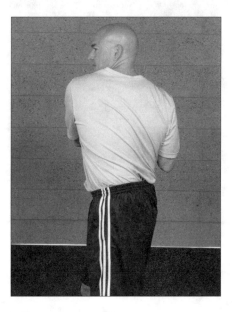

Comments and Tips

- This exercise should be performed as fast as possible while maintaining good technique. For top speed and good technique, the knees must be bent and the arms and upper body must move together.

- The shoulder-to-the-chin technique forces the emphasis on rotating the body evenly to each side as opposed to the arms moving without the shoulder turn.

The Chop

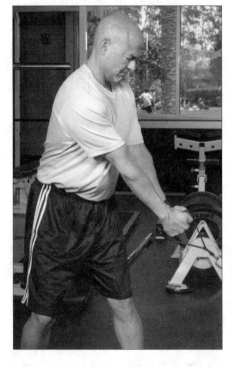 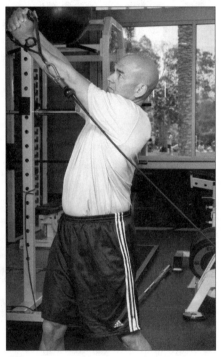

One-way chop—bottom Stand far enough from the cable so the arms are straight and the legs slightly bent. The shoulders should be positioned facing the cable so the hands and the middle of the chest are in line.

Tighten the midsection (abdominals and lower back) and rotate to bring the cable upward at approximately 45 degrees. Return to the starting position and repeat for the prescribed number of repetitions. Turn 180 degrees and repeat for the opposite side.

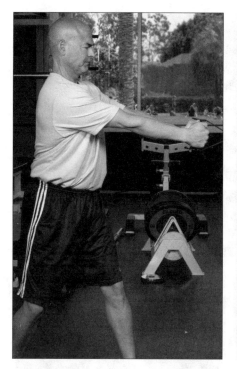 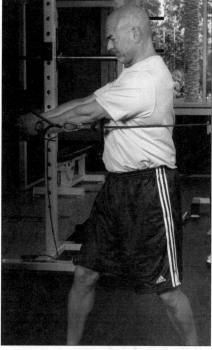

One-way chop—middle Again, stand far enough from the cable so the arms are straight and the legs are slightly bent. The shoulders are turned facing the cable and the grip is aligned with the middle of the chest.

After tightening the trunk, rotate while maintaining the shoulders/arms/hands relationship. Return to the starting position and repeat for the prescribed number of repetitions. Turn 180 degrees and repeat for the opposite side.

Comments and Tips

- A one-way chop is one of the three exercises, which would be designated top, middle, or bottom. A two-way chop would be any two of the three movements, and a three-way chop would be all three movements.

- Do not pivot on the back foot. The goal of the exercise is to make the trunk perform as much of the work as possible; when pivoting on the back foot, the hip is turned and this defeats the purpose of the exercise.

- Although the entire body forms a base of support, the point of the exercise is to rotate by using the abdominals only. One way to do this is to keep the arms straight (which is the biggest challenge in this exercise) and don't drive with the legs as you would in swinging a bat.

- Aside from the initial "pull," the weight stack should not touch during the exercise.

- Carefully choose the weight; a weight that is too heavy is not necessarily better and could cause injury.

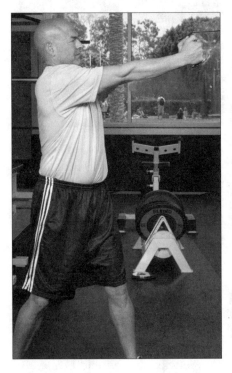

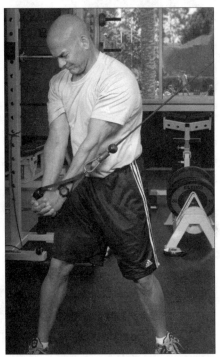

One-way chop—top To determine the distance from the cable, take the same stance as with the previous two movements.

After tightening the trunk, the cable is pulled downward by the body, not by the arms, at approximately 45 degrees. Return to the starting position and repeat for the prescribed number of repetitions. Turn 180 degrees and repeat for the opposite side.

Rotator Cuff Series

No baseball-training program would be comprehensive without paying attention to the rotator cuff of the shoulder. The supraspinatus, infraspinatus, teres minor, and subscapularis muscles make up the delicate and important rotator cuff. Without strength and fitness in this area, throwing a baseball with velocity and accuracy would be nearly impossible. A group of exercises performed 2–3 times per week will strengthen the rotator cuff. The following exercises—certainly not the only exercises available—should be performed as a warm-up to the weight-lifting program. While these exercises specifically train the "cuff," they also serve as an excellent all-around shoulder warm-up prior to upper body training.

Abducted External Rotation

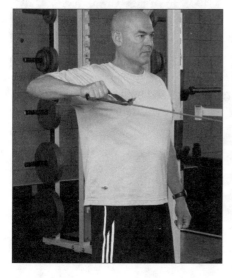
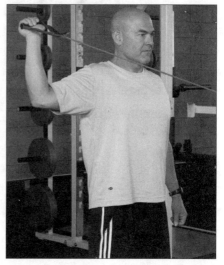

The tubing should be at the same height as the arm. Begin with the arm parallel to the ground, body upright and balanced, not leaning to one side or the other, and shoulders even. The elbow joint should be at 90 degrees.

Without any body movement or the use of additional musculature, maintain the height of the shoulder and bring the forearm to a position perpendicular to the ground. Be sure the movement is a deliberate and consistent motion. Lower and repeat. Should be performed with both arms.

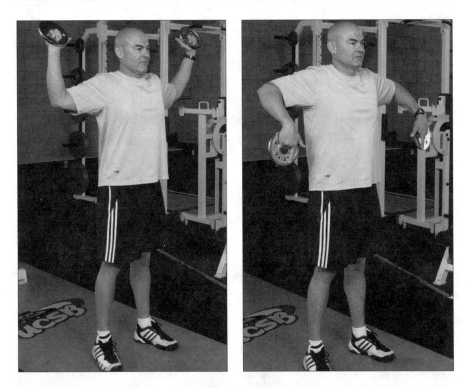

This exercise can also be performed with free weights and both arms simultaneously.

Adducted External Rotation

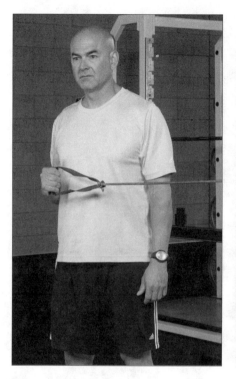 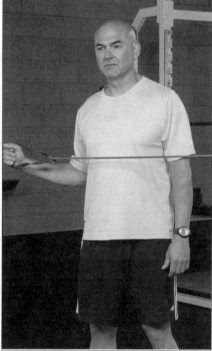

The upper arm is resting at the side of the body, forearm parallel to the ground, and the tubing is at the height of the forearm; the body is upright and balanced.

Without any body movement or the use of additional musculature, maintain the height of the forearm while moving the arm away from the body. Externally rotate as far as flexibility will allow; return to the starting position and repeat. To be performed with both arms.

Adducted Internal Rotation

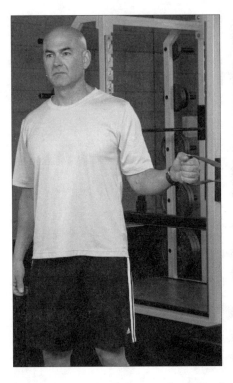 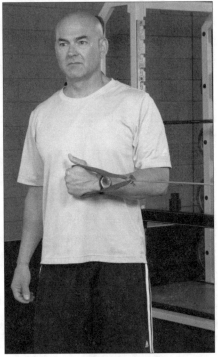

The upper arm is resting at the side of the body, the forearm parallel to the ground, and the tubing is at the height of the forearm; the body is upright and balanced. The elbow joint should be at 90 degrees.

Without any body movement or the use of additional musculature, maintain the height of the forearm while bringing the arm toward the midsection. Be sure the movement is a deliberate and consistent motion. To be performed with both arms.

Empty Can

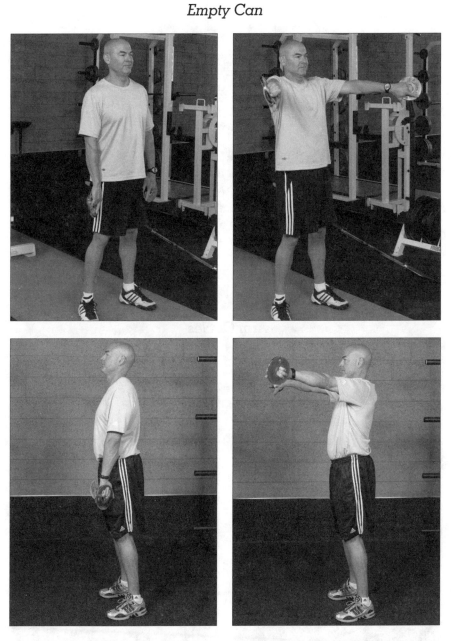

The arms should be at the side of the body with the thumbs touching the thighs.

Without shrugging the shoulders, raise the arms in a 45-degree path from the body to shoulder height. Maintain the thumbs-down position with the hand.

Comments and Tips

- Keep the shoulders from shrugging prior to raising the weight and during the exercise. A preliminary shrug usually means the weight is too heavy for the movement.

- Despite using a weight that would be considered very light, the movement should be performed with a rhythm of one second up and one second down.

Arm Circles

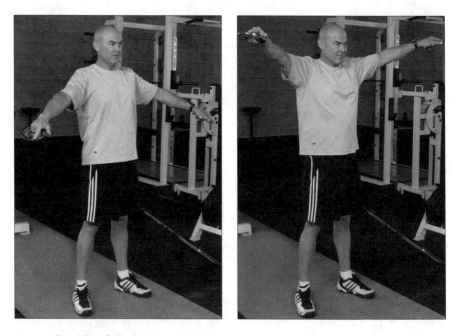

Out to the side of the body, rotate the arms in a small circle (12–24 inches in diameter) with a light weight (2–5 pounds), first clockwise and then counterclockwise.

CHANGING YOUR EXERCISE PROGRAM

As a program progresses, it might become necessary to add, delete, or substitute exercises. The core list should always remain the same, with changes occurring only when there is an injury, limitation, or significant strength or technical improvement. For example, one-leg squats would be substituted for back squats in the case of a lower-back injury. A one-leg squat would still emphasize the glutes, quadriceps, and hamstrings, but the significantly lighter load would be less stressful on the lower back.

An athlete can become "stale" if, while increasing strength or perfecting technique, additional or more challenging exercises are not added. In this case, the classic example is when an athlete's technique and strength is adequate enough to progress from the clean dead lift to the more advanced clean pulls. Also, with less trained or weaker athletes, it is sometimes necessary to begin with dumbbells in the bench press until enough strength is gained or technique is improved to proceed to the barbell bench press.

The most important point to remember when adding, substituting, or deleting exercises is to maintain a program balance in regards to over- or undertraining particular muscle groups. If additional front deltoid exercises are performed, then it is important to include additional rear deltoid exercises for shoulder balance. Likewise, deleting a hamstring exercise should lead to an increase in sets and/or repetitions in the remaining hamstring exercises and evaluating the exercise menu for the correct amount of quadriceps training. Always keep in mind that exercise menu modifications must also take into account the level of the athlete, training facility, and staff expertise.

5

Healthy Eating for Optimal Performance

Nutrition plays a critical role in athletic performance, but the problem is that many athletes do not eat a diet that helps them perform at their best. Do you approach every day knowing that the nutrients you are going to put into your body will enable you to perform at your best? Do you have a predetermined eating plan that is geared toward optimal performance? If you answered no to these questions, do not be discouraged. At this point, you are *ordinary*. This chapter is designed so that you will know what you need to eat on a daily basis. There are no tricks and no shortcuts, just the latest information designed to make you the best baseball player possible.

ENERGY REQUIREMENTS

Food is energy—to have enough energy, you need to consume enough food. Getting adequate calories from the right kinds of foods is what eating for optimal performance is all about. With too few calories, you will feel tired and weak and be more prone to injuries. By eating adequate calories from a variety of foods, you will satisfy your need for macronutrients (carbohydrates, protein, fat) and get the vitamins and minerals required for game-day performance.

Every individual has his own unique metabolism. This is obvious when you have two individuals who are the same weight but one of them eats significantly more calories than the other and does not gain weight. In order to determine how much food (calories) needs to be eaten on a daily basis, two pieces of information are needed: the resting energy expenditure and the activity factor. Resting energy expenditure is the fewest number of calories you need to eat on a daily basis. This does not include physical activity, such as resistance training and the energy that is expended during practice and games (this will be discussed under activity factor). To determine your resting energy expenditure, take your bodyweight (in pounds) and multiply by 11. For example, a 185-pound catcher can estimate resting energy expenditure by using this calculation: 185 x 11 = 2,035 calories. Then multiply this number (2,035 calories) by the appropriate activity factor. The activity factor is a number that estimates how many more calories you are expending each day as a result of lifestyle (type of occupation) and exercise (batting practice, conditioning drills, resistance training, etc.). To determine your activity factor, refer to Table 5.1. Most baseball players will have an activity factor of approximately 1.6. For our 185-pound catcher, whose resting energy expenditure is 2,035 calories and who has an activity factor of 1.6, this means that he should consume about 3,250 calories (2,035 x 1.6 = 3,256 calories).

TABLE 5.1 DETERMINING ACTIVITY FACTOR

LIFESTYLE AND EXERCISE LEVEL	ACTIVITY FACTOR
Resting—Sleeping; reclining	1.0
Sedentary—Watching television; reading	1.2
Light—Office work; walking	1.4
Moderate—Light manual labor; baseball; tennis	1.6
Very Active—Hard laborers; full-time athlete	1.9
Extremely Active—Full-time athletes with daily strenuous training	2.2

It is important to note that the values calculated for resting energy expenditure and activity factor are only estimates, and therefore are not absolute. It is up to you to apply these recommendations and then make any necessary adjustments for your particular situation. For instance, if you calculate how many calories you should be eating and discover that you are putting on too much body fat you will need to make adjustments.

Not a problem, as Chapter 7 deals with weight loss, and there you will find out exactly what to do to lose unwanted body fat.

WHAT TYPES OF FOODS TO EAT

Now that we have figured out how many calories to eat, you may be wondering how you are going to eat all of these calories and what types of foods you should be ingesting. It is very important to ingest 5–6 small meals throughout the day. In fact, this is so important that we will make it a rule. **Rule #1: Eat 5–6 meals per day.** Below is a description of not only the types of foods that should be eaten throughout the day, but also a plan for eating them in the correct combinations.

Carbohydrates

Carbohydrates are the main fuel that is burned during all intense activities. Hence, a diet focused primarily on *unprocessed* carbohydrates (i.e., fresh vegetables and fruits; stay away from packaged foods) is essential for players during all phases of training.

The basic source of energy for muscle contraction is adenosine triphosphate (ATP). The longer and more intense the muscular activity, as in a baseball game, the greater the need to rapidly supply ATP to your exercising muscles. The body relies on the phosphagen system, utilizing a substance called creatine phosphate to create more ATP. Since the primary energy system used for baseball is this phosphagen system (stored ATP and creatine phosphate), it is *not* necessary that you "load up" on carbohydrates. If you do that, you'll end up fatter than the third place guy at Nathan's hot dog eating contest.

Thus, the bulk of the day's calories—approximately 40 percent—should come from carbohydrates such as fresh fruits and vegetables. Try to limit your intake of white bread, bagels, pasta, and pizza; those are among your worst food choices. Your goal is to eat "clean" (lean meats, unprocessed carbohydrates, and healthy fats). Table 5.2 lists some great food choices that are rich in energy-producing carbohydrates. See Table 5.3 for the carbohydrates you should avoid.

Protein

Equally important to carbohydrate intake is protein intake. **Rule #2: Make sure each meal (5–6 meals per day) contains a source of protein.** Unlike carbohydrates, which are mainly a fuel source for anaerobic-type exercise, protein allows you to build and maintain muscle mass. The building and maintaining of muscle mass are two different but very important considerations for your nutrition program. The off-season is the time for building lean muscle mass and improving all-around conditioning. This can be accomplished via hard work in the weight room as well as proper nutrition and supplementation. During this phase of the off-season, protein intake is vital to your resistance-training program. In fact, we'd suggest that you *never* decrease protein intake! Protein should make up approximately 30 percent of the total calories consumed each day. A good estimate, based on body weight, is to consume about 1 gram of protein per pound of body weight (for a 200-pound player, this is equal to 200 grams of protein per day). Remember, it is important that protein is eaten at each meal, because if you allow several hours to elapse without eating protein, your body responds by breaking down your hard-earned muscle. For a list of foods that are good sources of protein, refer to Table 5.2. Table 5.3 lists unhealthy protein sources.

Fat

Fats are important for many metabolic processes, including energy production and as transporters of some vitamins. If carbohydrates make up 40 percent of the total calories and protein makes up an additional 30 percent, then the rest of the daily calories need to come from fats. This equates to approximately 30 percent. It is important to realize that not all fats are created equal. There are basically three types of fat found in foods: saturated fats, trans-fats, and unsaturated fats. Does this sound too technical? Don't worry, read on and soon you will be giving advice to the whole team in terms of what kinds of fats to eat and which ones to avoid.

For health reasons, you want to include more of the unsaturated fats from plant sources, such as nuts, olive and canola oils, and fatty fish like salmon and tuna. Trans-fatty acids (hydrogenated and partially hydrogenated fats) are associated with a number of health problems (remember, if you have poor health, you cannot perform to your capabilities). Trans-fats are artificial fats added to processed foods to increase shelf life. They are found in fried foods such as French fries, doughnuts, cookies, pastries, and crackers. An occasional meal containing these foods will not put an abrupt end to your baseball career, but make sure that foods containing trans-fats are not staples of your diet. See Table 5.2 for a list of healthy fats and Table 5.3 for the fats to avoid.

TABLE 5.2 HEALTHY FOOD CHOICES

CARBOHYDRATES	PROTEIN	FAT
Raw vegetables of all kinds	Fish	Fish fats
Fruit	Whole eggs (on occasion)	Nuts
Rice, preferably brown	Egg whites	Flax oil
Whole-grain bread	Milk, skim	Olive oil
Oatmeal	Whey meal replacement powders (MRPs)	
Beans	Casein MRPs	
Oatbran	Beef	
	Chicken	
	Pork	
	Soy	

TABLE 5.3 UNHEALTHY FOOD CHOICES

CARBOHYDRATES	PROTEIN	FAT
Anything with added sugar	Fatty meats	Butter
Anything with high-fructose corn syrup	Cold cuts	Margarine
Anything processed (which includes most things in the grocery aisles)	Processed meats of any kind	Foods with trans-fats
Regular bread		Fried food
Cereals		
Pasta		
Sodas (sugar filled)		
Candy		
Fruit juice		

Vitamins and Minerals

Vitamins and minerals do not contribute to energy directly, nor do they directly enhance strength and speed. However, fall short on consuming certain vitamins and minerals, and both energy production and muscle building will stop faster than a Nolan Ryan fastball in the catcher's mitt. The body cannot make vitamins and minerals; rather, they must be obtained from the foods that we eat. The great thing about following the recommendations given in this book—especially choosing the carbohydrates, proteins, and fats listed above—is that you will be eating foods full of the vitamins and minerals you need to perform optimally. As an insurance policy, we'd recommend that you also take a complete multivitamin/multimineral daily.

PREGAME, DURING GAME, AND POSTGAME NUTRITION—IT'S ALL ABOUT PERFORMANCE AND RECOVERY

Good nutrition is about more than what you eat—*when* you eat is equally important. New research indicates that what athletes eat before, during, and after a training session makes a big difference relative to performance and recovery. We will highlight not only what you should eat on game day, but also when you should eat it. Applying these nutritional techniques to game day will allow for the optimization of two important parameters—performance and recovery. Performance is manifested as speed, strength, power, and endurance. Optimal recovery allows you to repeat this high level of performance again very soon.

What good is it to inconsistently perform at an exceptionally high level? Many of the game's greatest athletes are a result of training and nutrition programs designed for optimal recovery. Why? Because they are able to recover from intense training sessions and games and come back refreshed the next day.

Recovery

Proper recovery allows you to come back from a previous bout of exercise or physical exertion so when you are called upon to perform again, you are able to do so in an optimal fashion. Conversely, if proper recovery is not attained, then subsequent training efforts (including actual game situations) are compromised for a variety of reasons. These compromises include improper muscle functioning, tissue injury, signs of overtraining, and decreases in immune function, all of which are detrimental to consistently performing at the highest level.

Although time and rest are critical to proper recovery, nutritional support is also an essential component. The best way to facilitate recovery (and optimal performance) from a nutritional perspective is to target the time periods associated with physical exertion. For our purposes, this is game day, and we will have a three-fold nutritional approach: pregame, during game, and postgame nutrition.

Pregame Nutrition

The primary purpose of pregame nutrition is to make sure you are mentally focused during the game. Let's face it, unless you're a pitcher, much of the time you spend during a game involves little to no movement. The primary energy system used by your body is stored ATP and creatine phosphate (the phosphagen energy system), so there is *no* need to load up on carbs. In fact, there's really no need to load up on any food! Your goal is to provide your body with just enough clean "fuel" so you are mentally alert. So, two or three hours pregame, it would be best to consume bland foods that contain low to moderate amounts of fats (you don't want to deal with digestive problems during the game) and have a small amount of protein and fibrous/starchy carbohydrates. Something like a half-cup of brown rice with a grilled chicken breast and a half-cup of broccoli would suffice. If you don't have time for a real meal, have a protein shake.

Nutrition During the Game

There are a few things to be aware of nutritionally during a game. If you are playing in high heat, drink fluids liberally to maintain normal hydration. This will prevent you from feeling tired. If you need a slight pick-me-up, we'd suggest low-dose caffeine (sip on an iced coffee drink with soy milk or low-fat milk and sugar-free sweetener). And don't worry about caffeine dehydrating you—that's just an urban legend.

What about sports drinks? Since you aren't moving much during a game, it is best to hydrate with water, not a sports drink. All the sports drink will do is feed you sugar. Consuming carbohydrates of any kind (e.g., sugar) can help restore muscle glycogen; however, glycogen depletion is *never* an issue in baseball. So if you're reaching for a sports drink, don't—reach for the H_2O instead.

Postgame Nutrition

The time period following a game is probably the most important time for nutritional intake. This is when recovery is critical and what you consume is of the utmost importance. Pizza and beer is a sure-fire way to get a fat gut. So be smart—the best source of replenishment postgame is a nutritious meal, one that contains carbohydrates, protein, electrolytes, and vitamins and minerals. As a matter of convenience, drink a protein shake immediately following a game, and then eat your normal meal an hour or so afterward.

More About Recovery

There is an old phrase that sports nutrition scientists have declared for years: "The three most important elements of training for optimal results are recovery, recovery, and recovery." This is what many nutritional strategies are designed for. Science has not shown conclusively that ingesting a pregame meal, a pregame snack, and a postgame beverage will improve specific skills needed for baseball. What we do know is that by following these nutritional tactics, you are allowing your body to recover from the stresses that intense activity produces. If not allowed to properly recover, your body cannot perform at an optimal level. Your brain will be telling your body one thing, but your body will not have the necessary nutrients to deliver the results that you demand of it.

These nutritional strategies are not solely for game day nutrition. Being fully recovered for the next game is very important, but you also want to be recovered for the next practice so you have the foundation on which to improve your skills. Therefore, apply these nutritional strategies on practice days and during spring training when conditioning drills are performed. By consistently addressing optimal recovery techniques through nutrition, you will be able to perform at your highest level at any point in the season.

CREATING THE PERFECT GAME DAY, NUTRITION-WISE

Now we will synthesize everything you have learned so far and put it into the perspective of a normal game day. In doing this, we assume two things: there is a game at 6:30 P.M., the game is an away game, and you will be traveling there by bus. If you are like the average baseball player on game day, you probably think that you just have to remember to bring your uniform and meet the team bus. As long as you do those two things, you will be prepared to play. Wrong! After reading this information, you will be thinking as an optimal performer should—you will begin to think about your food and water intake the night before the game! That's right, in order to eat for optimal performance and recovery, you must plan ahead. This means knowing what you are going to eat, preparing the food ahead of time, and having the necessary utensils to transport the prepared food when traveling (a small investment in plastic food storage containers goes a long way).

Planning Ahead

At this point, you know that you have to meet the team bus at 4 p.m., travel for an hour and a half, and then have one hour for warm-ups before the first pitch at 6:30 P.M. Because you are starting your nutritional and hydration plan the night before, you will guarantee you are adequately prepared and will be surprised at how easy it is to eat for optimal nutrition, as long as you plan ahead.

We established two rules in terms of eating for optimal performance: eat 5–6 meals per day, and make sure each meal eaten contains a source of protein. This will be the starting point. However, before determining what to eat, you have to determine when to eat. To do this, you have to take into consideration what time you will wake up, the time it will take traveling to the visitor's ballpark, and the amount of time the game will consume. Table 5.4 lists all of these variables, as well as the times designated for eating the meals you will prepare. Looking at the table, you may notice that you will be eating six times (Rule #1) and every meal is spaced out so you never allow more than three hours between each meal. This helps to ensure that you are not hungry and that your body has a constant supply of protein and other vital nutrients.

TABLE 5.4 PERFECT GAME DAY NUTRITION AND HYDRATION

SCHEDULE	FOOD	TOTAL CALORIES	CARBOHYDRATES-PROTEIN-FAT (%)	HYDRATION SCHEDULE
8:00 A.M. • *Wake Up*				
8:30 A.M. Meal 1	$^3/_4$ cup oatmeal 2 eggs (with $^1/_4$ cup of cheese) 16 oz. skim milk	650	40-25-35	Morning hours: Drink about 20 oz. of water between meals 1 and 2, and another 20 oz. between meals 2 and 3
11:30 A.M. Meal 2	6 oz. salmon $^1/_2$ cup carrots 1 apple Spinach salad (with $^1/_2$ oz. walnuts, dressing) 8 oz. orange juice	570	40-35-25	
2:30 P.M. Meal 3 (pregame meal)	Grilled chicken sandwich (whole-wheat bread with cheese, lettuce, tomato, onion) 1 cup broccoli 1 grapefruit 20 oz. water	660	40-35-25	
4 P.M. to 5:30 P.M. • *Travel to the Ballpark*				
Pregame (4:30 P.M. while traveling to the game)	Ingest about 17 oz. of water two hours before the start of the game			

TABLE 5.4 (continued)

Schedule	Food	Total Calories	Carbohydrates-Protein-Fat (%)	Hydration Schedule
5:30 P.M. Meal 4 (pregame snack)	2 nutrition bars (with adequate amounts of protein)	420	40-30-30	
6:30 P.M. to 9:00 P.M. • *Baseball Game*				
7:30 P.M. Meal 5 (during-game snack)	Sports nutrition beverage (sip occasionally; water is still better), *or,* Water or iced coffee (with sugar-free sweetener, soy milk) Attempt to ingest 4–8 oz. every 15–20 minutes; be more cognizant of this during warm weather play	320	65-35-0	
10:00 P.M. Meal 6 (post-game meal)	Protein shake, *or,* grilled chicken sandwich (with mayo, lettuce, tomato, onion); banana with 1 tbsp peanut butter, 20 oz. water	600	45-25-30	
Postgame:	Drink as needed as part of your post-game protein shake or with a meal			

Meal Composition

We will continue to use the example of a 185-pound catcher who requires approximately 3,250 calories. Also, remember that we want the majority of calories to come from carbohydrates (40 percent, more or less) and the rest to be approximately split between protein and fats (30 percent each). At this point, we know that we are going to eat six times on game day and that we want to consume about 3,250 calories throughout the day, and we know approximately how much carbohydrates, protein, and fat should comprise this amount. The only thing left to do is plan out the menu. Table 5.4 lists some options for the game-day scenario. It is important to note that these meals are not magical meals; they are just one example of many possible plans that would work well when eating for optimal performance and recovery on a game day.

If you focus on the total calories of each meal, you will notice that most of the calories are ingested during the earlier part of the day. This makes sense because you do not want your stomach to be full of food when you are about to perform any type of athletic endeavor. Also, by ingesting quality foods early on a game day, you can be confident that your body has time to digest and absorb all of the vital nutrients that it will need. In fact, the first three meals of the day comprise about 60 percent of the day's total calories.

Meals 1 and 2 both have a protein source (eggs, cheese, skim milk, salmon). Meal 1 has a good source of carbohydrate in the oatmeal, and meal 2 has a vegetable (carrots, spinach) and a fruit (apple, orange juice) for carbohydrates. We recommended that you try to include more unsaturated fats, and one of the best ways to do this is to eat more walnuts or other nuts (e.g., almonds). As you can see, there is a half-ounce serving of walnuts included in meal 2. Meal 3 provides more of the same quality nutrition: a protein source (grilled chicken), quality carbohydrate sources (whole-wheat bread, broccoli, and grapefruit), and a source of fat (cheese).

The Meals Before, During, and After the Game

So far in our game-day nutrition plan we have eaten only three meals, but we have also followed all of the rules set forth earlier. The next three meals will separate the winners from the losers in terms of proper meal planning. If you are not consistent in your nutritional planning, it will be most evident when you go on the road to play an away game.

Because meals 4 and 5 are smaller in terms of quantity and calories compared to the other meals, we define them as "snacks." But don't let this classification lessen the importance of these meals. While they are smaller in total calories, they are just as important in our nutritional strategy. Meal 4 (pregame snack) should be eaten about an hour before the game. In this case of an away game, it should be ingested when the team arrives at its destination and right before warm-ups. Table 5.4 lists two nutrition bars for this meal; they travel easily and usually contain adequate amounts of protein. If you prefer not to eat nutrition bars, then a banana with peanut butter or a container of yogurt with some fruit are great alternatives. Meal 5 (during-game snack) is to be consumed during the game. Because of the importance of maintaining proper hydration levels, a sports nutrition beverage that contains plenty of water and some carbohydrates and protein would be ideal at this time. Notice that this meal contains no fat. This omission is purposeful, for fat takes longer to digest than carbohydrates and protein. For this reason, you want to keep fat intake low during competition.

By the time the game is over, your nutritional strategies have helped you perform well on the field. However, the team will be stopping at a fast food restaurant on the way home. Now what do you do? You have eaten perfectly all day, you have followed your plan, and now you will be forced to eat fast food. Is all lost? Not at all. There are almost always healthy and proper food choices at all restaurants—you just have to know what they are. Meal 6 (postgame meal) lists a grilled chicken sandwich, but is this a good choice? You have eaten only five meals so far, and you know that in order to properly recover, you need to eat after every game, practice, or workout. Consequently, if you are thinking that you need to eat *something,* you are correct. Does this meal contain a source of protein? Sure, the grilled chicken. In addition to that, the bun contains carbohydrates, and you are going to drink 20 ounces of water with it to assist in rehydration. Also, because you planned ahead and packed a banana and peanut butter, you have added a quality carbohydrate in the form of a fruit and some healthy unsaturated fats with the peanut butter. Overall, not a bad result for a fast food meal and a little bit of planning.

Water and Hydration

Our game-day nutrition plan only has 40 ounces of water (during meals 3 and 6) listed throughout the entire day. Even though skim milk and orange juice contain a lot of water, this is still not enough water intake for optimal performance. In addition to these beverages, Table 5.4 on page 108 lists a hydration schedule for the entire day.

Putting It All Together

At the end of the day, this nutritional plan supplies approximately 3,220 calories with a macronutrient breakdown of 45 percent carbohydrates, 30 percent protein, and 25 percent fat. Not only were six meals eaten (Rule #1), but each meal contained a source of protein (Rule #2) and quality carbohydrates. Adequate planning before, during, and after the game allowed the nutritional plan to become a reality, even while traveling for an away game. It is this type of *consistent* planning and execution that will allow you to perform at your best.

Recall that we wanted to plan a daily caloric intake of 3,250 calories for our hypothetical 185-pound catcher. Also, we wanted the calories to be divided into 40 percent carbohydrates, 30 percent protein, and 30 percent fat. You may be asking if we have failed in our goals after all—our game day diet only supplied 3,220 calories (30 calories less than desired) and our caloric breakdown was not exact either. These slight differences are not anything to stress over. Do not get overwhelmed in making sure that each meal is *exactly* perfect in terms of total calories and macronutrient breakdown. If you do this, you will spend more time planning each meal than you will practicing baseball drills. Rather, just follow the guidelines set forth in this chapter:

- Eat 5–6 meals per day.

- Make sure each meal contains a source of protein.

- Derive a majority of your carbohydrates from fruit and vegetables.

- Include unsaturated fats (from nuts, oils, and fish) in your diet.

- Stay well hydrated.

6

Supplements to Enhance Baseball Performance

In this chapter, we will present the latest information on supplements that may assist you in your baseball performance goals. It must be stated that these supplements are not a replacement for adequate nutrition. It is best to follow a great nutritional regimen and a supplementation scheme in order to achieve optimal performance in any sport.

In order to properly choose a supplement that may improve your performance on the diamond, you first must realize what types of physiological constraints limit baseball performance. Baseball requires athletes to possess quick reflexes, explosive power, an ability to quickly accelerate and decelerate, and an ability to recover from maximal exertion. The sports supplements outlined here have been shown to positively affect these key areas.

Before you start taking any of these supplements, it is very important that you first consult with a sports nutrition scientist (for more information, go to the website of the International Society of Sports Nutrition at www.theissn.org). Secondly, check with your governing organization or league (MLB, NCAA, high school associations, etc.) regarding their stance on supplementation. Also, be sure to follow the recommended dosages for each supplement that you take.

CREATINE MONOHYDRATE

Of all the supplements recommended, creatine monohydrate is by far the most researched and proven to be safe and effective. Study after study has demonstrated that creatine will enhance muscular power and muscular strength, and improve recovery from maximal exertion. Baseball is purely an anaerobic sport—all of the movements in baseball are centered on short-term (a few seconds) high-intensity activities. Coincidentally, creatine supplementation leads to significant improvements in short-term, intense exercise performance, which makes creatine perfect for improving baseball performance. In addition to improving short-term sprinting performance and recovery, creatine supplementation leads to gains in body mass of about 2–5 pounds, mostly as lean body mass. Also, creatine supplementation will make you stronger in the weight room.

Many sports nutritionists would argue that creatine is the single most important discovery in the history of sports supplementation, particularly because muscle creatine stores can be elevated by oral ingestion of the dietary supplement. Creatine, or methylguanidine-acetic acid, is naturally produced in your body from the amino acids methionine, arginine, and glycine (which are essential, conditionally essential, and nonessential amino acids, respectively).

In one study of creatine, 31 male subjects were tested for muscle creatine levels, creatine degradation, and creatinine excretion when consuming either 20 grams (g) or 3 g of creatine per day for 28 days. The researchers found that total muscle creatine concentrations increased by 20 percent after the first six days of supplementation with the 20 g load. However, the same 20 percent increase was noted after 28 days of consuming the 3 g dose—the increase simply occurred more gradually. Other studies have found that subjects consuming creatine at a level of 0.1 g/kg/lean body mass/day (about 6–8 g per day) excreted approximately half of the ingested dose (about 3–4 g) and the rest was absorbed into muscle. It has been reported that a maintenance dose of just 2 g per day for 30 days was effective at maintaining an elevated level of total muscle creatine. A 2 g dose that maintains elevated muscle creatine levels may not, however, continue to maintain improvements in performance. For example, when handball players received a loading dose of 15 g/day for five days, tests measuring repeated 40-meter sprints improved. After the loading phase, a 2 g daily dose was employed for the following nine days. The researchers noted that although sprint times in later trials were still significantly better than before supplementation with creatine, there was no continued improvement.

However, if you currently do not take creatine and want to quickly improve muscle power and strength, then loading clearly does work. For instance, one study showed that three days of creatine supplementation can increase thigh muscle volume and may enhance cycle sprint performance in elite power athletes; additionally, this effect is greater in females as sprints are repeated.

Regarding dosages of creatine, you can take one of two approaches. The first approach is recommended if you want to saturate your muscles with creatine in the shortest amount of time possible. In this situation, it is recommended to orally ingest 5 grams (g) of creatine four times daily (for a daily total of 20 g) for five days. After this five-day loading period, you can decrease the dosages to 3 g once a day. Alternatively, if you have no need for immediate creatine saturation, studies have shown that ingesting 3 g of creatine for 30 days results in similar levels of creatine saturation inside the muscles. These two alternatives for creatine supplementation are important. The occasional and haphazard supplementation of creatine before some practices and games will not result in any type of performance enhancement. Rather, consistent supplementation day after day is the only way creatine will result in improved game-day and practice performance.

In the past few years, there have been many media reports about the horrors of creatine supplementation. This type of reporting on creatine has been either misguided or intentionally misleading. The fact is that creatine supplementation is safe and effective. In fact, the only consistently reported side effect associated with creatine supplementation is weight gain, and this is in the form of lean muscle mass! Another common media story about creatine supplementation is that we do not know the *long-term* side effects. The truth is that creatine has been researched in clinical trials ranging from several years to nearly 20 years with no reported adverse effects.

All of the available evidence about creatine supplementation leads us to believe that it may be an effective means to improve baseball performance for some players. However, there are some individuals who do not seem to benefit from creatine. For these individuals, some of the other supplements discussed in this chapter may be beneficial. For those individuals who benefit from creatine, it not only improves performance during games but it also may lead to increases in strength and recovery during the off-season. A stronger athlete and one who is better recovered will have more productive practices and will ultimately be able to perform at higher levels of competition on a consistent basis. In this regard, creatine supplementation should be used to increase the intensity and productivity of the practices that are conducted in the off-season and on nongame days. Remember, if your individual practices are of high quality, then your game performance will reflect this.

BETA-ALANINE

Beta-alanine is a new supplement with few studies investigating its potential. It may best serve as a training aid. The few studies that have been conducted all point to this novel compound as a performance enhancer. Beta-alanine works by increasing muscular levels of a compound known as carnosine. (Just ingesting carnosine is not an efficient way of accomplishing this.) Carnosine (beta-alanyly-L-histidine), composed of two amino acids, histidine and beta-alanine, may help slow the build-up of acids in the muscles during exertion, thus allowing you to work longer and harder.

Research has shown that beta-alanine combined with creatine improves performance, particularly short-term, all-out maximal exertion exercise. For instance, a recent study looked at the effect of beta-alanine alone or in combination with creatine monohydrate on aerobic exercise performance. Fifty-five men (average age of 24.5 years) participated in a double-blind, placebo-controlled study and were randomly assigned to one of four groups: placebo, creatine, beta-alanine, or beta-alanine plus creatine. According to the authors, the combination of supplements may enhance endurance-type performance. Recently, a study in mice looked at supplementation with beta-alanine in drinking water for one week. Beta-alanine intake reduced liver taurine levels, but elevated cysteine levels significantly. Therefore, the enhanced availability of cysteine for synthesis of glutathione and/or taurine appears to account for the protective effects of beta-alanine against liver injury. Thus, beta-alanine by itself has an ergogenic effect and may also have an antioxidant effect in the liver.

Most of the studies that have looked at beta-alanine supplementation have used dosages in the range of 3–6 g per day. Currently, many sports supplement companies are combining creatine with beta-alanine into one product. Even though the research is limited, it appears that this combination would be beneficial for baseball players. A dose of 3–6 g daily is needed to get an ergogenic effect (enhances physical performance). Also, you need to be on the supplement for at least 4–6 weeks prior to seeing such an effect.

CAFFEINE

Cognitive function is a fancy term for how well the brain is functioning. Before you can begin to get the bat around on an 90-mile-per-hour fastball, your brain first has to process these factors: estimate how fast the ball is coming, determine the trajectory of the ball, decide to not only swing the bat but also at what plane you should start your swing, select how fast to swing, determine the time at which you should rotate your hips, and so on. The point is that your brain must not only factor in all of these variables, but also must communicate these stimuli to the correct muscles at the correct times in order for an athletic movement to result in success. Because baseball is a sport that relies on quick reflexes and instant body positioning (both at the plate and while making defensive plays in the field), it makes sense that any ergogenic aid that enhances these components may be worth its weight in gold. Caffeine may be just the supplement to address these components of baseball performance. In some individuals, caffeine improves alertness, concentration, reaction time, and energy levels. Each one of these effects should theoretically improve baseball performance.

Caffeine, however, does have a multitude of other effects (besides enhancing mental function). These include enhanced metabolic rate and increased utilization of fat as a fuel, and there is a huge volume of data showing that it enhances performance. Caffeine can ratchet up your body's furnace so you burn more calories. An oft-used technique by fitness competitors is to down a strong cup of coffee or a caffeine pill prior to exercise. You'll exercise harder, longer, and burn more fat in the process.

Have a Cup of Joe

There's nothing better than a great cup of coffee first thing in the morning while you read the newspaper. In fact, more than 100 million Americans make a beeline for the coffee brewer, with eyes half open and joints slightly stiff. It is the caffeine in coffee that produces the myriad benefits many seek.

Caffeine Content in Beverages

Beverage	Serving	Caffeine Dose
Fortified coffee	8 oz	~300 mg
Coffee	1 cup	~60–150 mg
Cola drinks	12 oz can	~40 mg
Tea	1 cup	~20–50 mg
Hot cocoa	1 cup	~6 mg
Decaffeinated coffee	1 cup	~2–5 mg

Consuming coffee can have myriad health benefits, including increased mental and physical performance, enhanced fat burning, and an improvement in health.

- Coffee may decrease the risk of oral/pharyngeal, esophageal, and colorectal cancers.
- Long-term coffee consumption decreases your risk for type 2 diabetes.
- Coffee drinking is associated with reduced risk of alcohol-associated pancreatitis and liver disease.
- There is no association between coffee intake and risk of pancreatic cancer or rheumatoid arthritis.
- Increased coffee consumption was associated with a decreased risk of invasive epithelial ovarian cancer (EOC).
- Coffee drinking does not increase the risk of coronary heart disease or breast cancer incidence.

What about for baseball? On hot days, a great solution is iced coffee. On cold days, drink it hot. It'll give you a helpful energy boost.

A recent study looked at energy expenditure, fat oxidation (burning), and norepinephrine kinetics (i.e., how adrenaline-like hormones are metabolized) after caffeine or placebo ingestion. They studied ten older (65–80 years old) and ten younger (19–26 years old) men who were moderate consumers of caffeine. The dose administered was 5 mg of caffeine per kilogram of fat-free mass (which is mainly muscle and bone). The younger men consumed about 350 mg while the older men consumed about 295 mg. Caffeine ingestion resulted in similar increases in both the older and younger men for plasma caffeine levels. Metabolic rate or energy expenditure increased by 11 percent in the young men and 9.5 percent in the older men. Thus, older and younger men showed a similar thermogenic response to caffeine, whereas older men showed a smaller increase in fatty acid availability after caffeine. The differences were not related to alterations in norepinephrine kinetics or fat oxidation. Caffeine is a great ergogenic aid that promotes fat metabolism, improves performance, and ratchets up your metabolic rate.

Common caffeine dosages range from 1.5–3.0 milligrams (mg) daily per pound of bodyweight (approximately 250–525 mg of caffeine for a 175-pound individual). While side effects are rare, individuals who take more than the recommended dosages may experience nervousness, anxiety, insomnia, and shaking hands. Also, caffeine consumption does not dehydrate you, despite the commonly heard notion that it does. At least that's what the science says.

MISCELLANEOUS SUPPLEMENTS

The following supplements are included because there is enough scientific evidence to conclude they may indirectly improve performance via increases in lean body mass or an improvement in overall body composition. Theoretically, a lean, muscular baseball player should perform better than his or her fat counterpart.

Leucine and the Essential Amino Acids (EEAs)

There is a growing body of evidence that leucine, an essential amino acid and one of the branched-chain amino acids (BCAAs, the others are valine and isoleucine) can improve performance and promote gains in lean body mass. A recent study looked at the effects of dietary leucine supplementation on the exercise performance of outrigger canoeists. Thirteen (ten female and three male) competitive outrigger canoeists underwent testing before and after six-week supplementation with either L-leucine (45 mg/kg body weight) or a placebo. Upper body power and work significantly increased in both groups after supplementation, but power was significantly greater after leucine supplementation compared to the placebo. Rowing time significantly increased and average RPE (ratings of perceived exertion) significantly decreased with leucine, while these variables were unchanged with the placebo.

Scientists know that both insulin and leucine are key regulators in muscle protein synthesis. And leucine by itself increases muscle protein synthesis. By combining leucine with proteins and carbohydrates, you get an anabolic super-effect. For example, in one study, eight male subjects were randomly assigned to three trials in which they consumed drinks containing either carbohydrate (CHO), carbohydrate and protein (CHO+PRO), or carbohydrate, protein, and free leucine (CHO+PRO+Leu) following 45 minutes of resistance exercise. Plasma insulin response was highest in the group given leucine. Whole-body protein breakdown rates were lower, and whole-body protein synthesis was higher, in the CHO+PRO and CHO+PRO+Leu trials. Moreover, the addition of leucine resulted in a lower protein oxidation rate. Muscle protein synthesis, measured over a six-hour period of postexercise recovery, was significantly greater in the leucine trial.

So should you supplement with leucine? It certainly could help, but an even better option may be to supplement with all of the essential amino acids (EAAs). A recent study looked at alterations of the acute hormonal response associated with liquid carbohydrate and/or EAA ingestion on hormonal and muscular adaptations following resistance training. Thirty-two untrained young men performed 12 weeks of resistance training (twice a week), consuming either a 6 percent carbohydrate solution (approximately 675 ml), an EAA mixture (6 g), a combination supplement, or a placebo. Muscle fiber size increased the most in the combination group. Thus, the combination of carbohydrates and the essential amino acids is perhaps the best way of promoting gains in lean body mass.

Protein

Previously, we suggested that each meal should include some source of protein. Admittedly, this can be difficult to achieve in some circumstances, which is why we recommend protein supplements. Over the last fifteen years, there have been significant advances in the development of these supplements. Today, there are numerous protein supplements that supply high-quality protein and also taste delicious. These supplements are available in liquid, powder, or bar form. By using protein supplements, you can make sure you consume protein 5–6 times a day without a problem. This enables your body to increase or maintain muscle mass as well as muscular strength.

In one study, scientists looked at the effects of ten weeks of resistance training and protein supplementation on muscle performance and markers of muscle anabolism. Nineteen untrained males were randomly assigned to two supplement groups, including placebo or protein. At each exercise session participants were provided their respective supplement, mixed with 500 ml of water, one hour before and immediately after exercise. The placebo group received a total of 40 g of dextrose, whereas the protein group received a total of 40 g of protein (14 g whey protein concentrate, 6 g whey protein isolate, 4 g milk protein isolate, 4 g calcium caseinate, and 12 g of free amino acids). Both supplements had the same number of calories. On nonexercise days, 40 g of the placebo or protein was ingested in the morning upon waking. Participants exercised four times per week (three sets of 6–8 repetitions at 85–90 percent of the one repetition maximum).

What happened? The protein supplement resulted in greater increases in total body mass, fat-free mass, thigh mass, muscle strength, and myofibrillar (muscle) protein. The fact that the protein supplement was better than a carbohydrate placebo, despite less of an insulin response, may have been due to the added free amino acids, especially the 6 g leucine. So in a sense, insulin is only part of the equation. Other factors such as IGF-1 (a type of growth factor) and the concentrations of EAAs in your blood are other determinants of the anabolic response. For you carbohydrate addicts, this study shows the futility of loading up on carbs. This study supports others showing that in the battle of protein versus carbs, protein wins without breaking a sweat.

When shopping for a protein supplement, look for one that contains whey, casein, or a combination of these two proteins. Both of these proteins are relatively inexpensive and contain all of the essential amino acids that your body needs to synthesize and maintain muscle.

Vitamins and Minerals

Vitamins do not directly provide energy or increase muscle mass, but they do provide functions that are critical for normal energy metabolism. The best sources of vitamins are fruits and vegetables, and we have repeatedly recommended throughout this book the importance of eating these types of foods every day. That being said, in reality, few individuals eat perfectly every day of their lives. For this reason, we recommend a quality multivitamin with minerals. Your home-to-first time may not improve from doing this, but it will serve to offset poor eating and may offer other health benefits (for example, vitamin E has both cancer-fighting properties and improves the health of blood vessels).

Glucosamine

Glucosamine is important for joint health. While all athletes need to take care of their joints, if you are a catcher or pitcher, glucosamine supplementation is highly recommended. Glucosamine not only will help repair injured joints, but it may help prevent joint injuries from occurring. How many baseball careers have ended because of elbow, shoulder, knee, or lower back problems? Too many to name. Hence, doing everything you can to help maintain the structure and integrity of your joints is a wise decision if you want to be playing for years to come. Common forms of glucosamine supplements are glucosamine sulfate and glucosamine chondroitin. Either one of these are good choices for preventing or repairing previous joint problems. A dose of 1,500 mg of glucosamine daily may be worth trying.

Glutamine

The amino acid glutamine has a broad range of potential benefits. Not only does glutamine support your immune system, it also prevents muscle loss and enhances recovery. Glutamine supplementation becomes more of a necessity when the intensity of your training is high or when the frequency of games increases during the season. These circumstances often lead to overtraining. Signs of overtraining are lethargy, decreases in strength, and suppression of the immune system. Glutamine has the potential to help offset these negative consequences. The easiest way to consume glutamine is postworkout at a dose of 5–15 g.

Essential Fatty Acids

If you're on a low-fat diet, don't be. You need dietary fat, especially the essential fatty acids. The word *essential* means that the body is not capable of producing these necessary fats, and the only way to obtain them is from certain foods (such as nuts, olive and canola oil, and fatty fish like salmon and tuna) or through essential fatty acid supplements. Since it is not always convenient to cook fish or add oils to certain meals, an essential fatty acid supplement is highly recommended. Supplements that contain these essential fatty acids include borage oil, flax seed oil, and fish oil supplements. Coincidentally, essential fatty acids are not only beneficial for general health, they also contribute to optimal joint health. If you don't consume much fat, consume flax oil or fish oil capsules.

7

Weight Loss and Weight Gain— The Right Way

WEIGHT LOSS STRATEGIES

Many individuals embark on a weight loss program in the wrong way. They employ methods that not only do not work in the long term but also cause their athletic performance to nose-dive. In some instances, the weight loss strategies employed can be downright harmful. When attempting to lose weight, you really only want to lose body fat. The last thing you want is to lose lean body mass (muscle). Muscle is hard enough to maintain and even harder to build, so why would you want to commit nutritional suicide and lose this precious tissue? It may be difficult to lose body fat without any concomitant losses in muscle, but it can be done. Even if some muscle mass is lost while attempting to lose weight, it is our goal to minimize this.

This concept is so important that we need to have a safeguard to make sure that the weight lost is not primarily lean body mass. The most effective way to do this is to have your body composition measured every few weeks while attempting to lose weight. A body composition assessment measures how much of your total body weight is comprised of fat and how much is comprised of muscle. Most health clubs offer body composition assessments as part of their services, but you can also purchase body-weight scales that estimate body composition or purchase skin calipers that do the same thing. If, after following the advice in this chapter, you find yourself ten pounds lighter, and a body composition measurement has revealed that nine pounds of it was from body fat, then you are right on track. As a rule of thumb, it is always best to minimize lean body mass loss. This can be accomplished by *never* decreasing your protein intake. In fact, it is recommended that you keep your protein intake fairly high at all times (i.e., 1 gram of protein daily per pound of body weight). Otherwise, you will find yourself on the bench real quick, and if you are not careful, a slight wind will take you with it!

The most effective approach to weight loss involves a regimen that offers a slight reduction in caloric intake, the replacement of processed carbohydrates with protein or unsaturated fat, and an increase in the amount of calories that are burned through exercise. Because you are an athlete and are already physically active, reducing caloric intake may play a larger role in your weight loss goals than does increasing physical activity. However, we do have a few exercise tricks that will not only assist you in your weight loss goals, but can actually improve your baseball performance. Exactly how much exercise and how many calories to cut are going to be individualized, but by following these guidelines you can be confident that you are on the right path.

Reduce Calories and Manipulate Macronutrients

Many weight loss experts suggest that the best way to lose weight is via a slight reduction in total daily calories combined with a replacement of processed carbohydrates (e.g., breads, pasta, pastries) with protein or unsaturated fat. We recommend that you start by reducing your caloric intake by 250 calories per day. What is the best way to delete these calories from your diet? Is it to decrease your meals to only four per day? Absolutely not—this would violate Rule #1 (eat 5–6 meals per day). The best way to reduce your calories is by reducing the total amount of calories by a small amount from each meal.

Or just reduce your intake of simple sugars or processed carbohydrates. In Chapter 5, we recommended that your daily calories be divided into 40 percent carbohydrates, 30 percent protein, and 30 percent fat. Reducing your carbohydrates slightly may lead to faster fat loss. If you decide to reduce your carbohydrates during your weight loss program, we recommend dropping them to 33 percent of your total daily calories.

Attempt to obtain the rest of your calories from an equal amount of protein and fat (33 percent each).

As a general guideline, an acceptable rate of weight loss should be no more than two pounds per week. If weight is lost faster than this, chances are that lean body mass is being sacrificed. In addition to frequent measurements of body composition, use this two-pound maximum to gauge your progress.

Exercise More

Increased energy expenditure via training is the other side of the weight loss coin. In addition to your already designed program, extra drills that are recommended include extra baserunning drills, outfield work (running down fly balls, etc.), or infield work (fielding ground balls). Certainly, your strength-and-conditioning coach can work with you in being creative about your exercise selection. Any baseball-related drill kills two birds with one stone: performing these drills an extra 30 minutes per day expends at least 200 calories and improves your game at the same time. These types of drills are only a few of the many examples that could be performed to assist in burning additional calories.

Fat Loss Supplements

Fat loss supplements work in three main ways: reduce appetite (suppress hunger), help burn fat, or block fat storage. One thing fat loss supplements cannot do is magically reduce weight without any effort on your part. The following fat loss supplements should only be tried if you are already reducing your caloric intake and performing additional baseball-specific conditioning drills. These are truly "supplements" to an effective fat loss nutrition plan and extra baseball conditioning drills.

Caffeine is one of the most commonly used ingredients in fat loss supplements. It works by stimulating the central nervous system and increasing the rate at which your body burns fat. Combined with exercise, caffeine can add a real boost to your fat loss. The nice thing about this supplement is that it is found in abundance in coffee and tea, so if you enjoy these beverages, feel free to include them in your nutritional plan for weight loss.

Green tea is another healthy beverage that may help you lose weight. In addition to the liquid tea form, it can also be taken as a supplement. Like caffeine, green tea causes an increase in the rate at which fat is burned. Interestingly, it appears that when green tea is combined with caffeine, the amount of calories burned is greater than when either of these supplements is ingested alone.

Because many individuals have great difficulty dealing with the resulting hunger that comes from decreasing calories, appetite suppressants have been marketed as a method of dealing with this problem. Because many of these supplements have not been shown to be effective for weight loss, we do not recommend them. Protein produces more of a feeling of fullness than carbohydrates and fats. In this regard, protein can be regarded as an appetite suppressant. If you have been a good student and always include a source of protein in each of your meals, congratulations! You have been employing a secret weapon to assist you in your weight loss goals. Either way, these supplements should not serve as a substitute for clean eating and hard exercise.

Summary of Weight Loss Recommendations

Many individuals fail in their attempts to lose weight. Even when successful at losing weight, many individuals lose too much lean body mass, which we define as failure. Remember, the ultimate goal when attempting to lose weight is to lose as much body fat as possible and to maintain lean body mass. Follow these guidelines to achieve this goal:

- Initially, reduce caloric intake by 250–500 calories per day and make adjustments as necessary.

- Lose no more than two pounds per week.

- Reduce carbohydrate (especially processed carbs) intake and replace it with lean protein and healthy fats.

- Supplementation and frequent protein intake may improve the amount and rate of fat loss.

- Obtain regular (at least once per month) body composition assessments.

STRATEGIES FOR GAINING LEAN BODY MASS

Sports scientists have been researching how to gain muscle for many years, and they have come to the conclusion that only two things actually work for putting on lean body mass: intense resistance training and proper nutrition. These two ingredients are not only essential for muscle-building success, they also must complement each other before ideal lean body mass can be achieved.

When attempting to gain lean body mass, patience is the key. Even if you do everything perfectly (meaning that you follow the advice given in this chapter), it will still take several months before you will visibly see any gains in lean body mass. This is often frustrating for the ordinary ballplayer who sets out to gain muscle mass. You must dedicate yourself to do what it takes—day after day, week after week, and month after month. Just remember that it will take time to see changes in your physique, but if you are consistent, you will be very satisfied with the results. Our discussion of gaining lean body mass will begin with the most important piece of this puzzle—a proper resistance training program.

Training for Lean Body Mass

Spending time in the weight room is a must if you are to increase lean body mass. Since you are training to improve your performance in baseball, you will have to balance your weight room training with your other baseball-specific drills and conditioning, being careful to not overtrain. When designing a resistance training program, you need to address these five things:

- How many days per week of training you are able to perform
- Exercises to include in the program
- Number of sets for each exercise
- Number of repetitions (reps) per set
- Rest time between sets

The best way to gain lean body mass is to train the entire body, because this allows many muscles to hypertrophy (get bigger). For the sake of simplicity, let's divide your body into lower body muscle groups and upper body muscle groups. Lower body muscles include glutes, quadriceps, hamstrings, abductors (the muscles on the outside of your thighs), adductors (the muscles on the inside of your thighs), and calves. Upper body muscles include back, chest, abdominals, shoulders, biceps, triceps, and forearms.

Frequency

Next, you have to determine the *frequency* of your workouts, or how many days per week you wish to train these body parts. This is where some delicate planning on your part must come into play. We recommend splitting whole body training into 3–6 days per week, training separate groupings of body parts on each day. During the baseball season, training six days per week is not recommended because you would not want to train legs or shoulders on the day of a game. While you may be building muscle, you may not have enough time to recover adequately and hence may not be able to perform optimally on the field. On the other hand, in the off-season, you may be able to do resistance training six days per week without worrying about having a game on the same days as intense training sessions.

For our purposes, we will outline an off-season workout under the assumption that you have decided to train four days per week. The goal is to make sure that you train each body part one time per week. The table on the following page shows a weekly training split that accomplishes this, as well as listing some exercises that are excellent for targeting each body part. Notice that the training days generally alternate between the lower body and the upper body—this type of training split has been shown to be effective and is commonly used.

These exercises should be performed for 3–5 sets of 6–12 repetitions. (This program could be used year round in order to promote muscle gain.) The table gives specific days for training specific body parts, but this is not a magical training program. You will need to experiment with many different regimens and training days to see what works best for you. The only thing that you must do is be consistent with the resistance training program that you have chosen.

LEAN BODY MASS OFF-SEASON TRAINING SPLIT		
DAY	**MUSCLE GROUP**	**POSSIBLE EXERCISES**
Monday	Quads, Glutes, Adductors	Squats, Leg Extensions, One-Leg Squat
Tuesday	Chest, Triceps, Forearms, Abdominals	Bench Press, Incline Barbell Bench Press, Tricep Push Down, Hammer, Gripper, Three-Way Chop
Wednesday	Off	
Thursday	Hamstrings, Abductors, Shoulders	Leg Curls, Bent-Leg Dead Lift with Barbell, Dumbbell Shrug, Two-Arm Dumbbell Lateral Raise, Two-Arm Bent Lateral Raise
Friday	Back, Biceps, Abdominals	Two-Arm Lat Pull Down, Seated Cable Row, One-Arm Lat Pull Down, Barbell Curls, Seated Twist, Lying Twist
Saturday	Off	
Sunday	Off	

Sets, Reps, and Rest Periods

Commonly recommended set and rep schemes are 3–5 sets of 6–12 reps. What this means is that you want to select a weight (resistance) for a given exercise so you are able to do at least six repetitions and no more than twelve repetitions per set. If you are unable to perform six reps, then you need to lower the weight until you have built up enough strength to handle the recommended set and rep ranges. In relation to rest periods between sets, we recommend that you rest long enough to fully recover from the previous set. This will usually be about two minutes of rest between each set, but it can vary based on the muscle group (quads and glutes may require more rest than biceps and forearms). Again, you will need to experiment and keep good notes as to what your ideal rest periods should be.

Periodization and Progression

There are several proven fundamentals that result in increases in lean body mass. One of these is known as periodization, a fancy word for changing your resistance training routine often. This can be done by learning new exercises, changing the order of your exercises, adding or deleting some sets during your routine, changing up which body parts are trained on certain days, and even changing the rest periods. Basically, you do not want to be doing the same resistance training program one year from now. Your body becomes accustomed to certain movements and actually becomes so efficient that it no longer responds as favorably to exercises that are repeated over and over. Conversely, if you keep alternating and changing things in your routine, your body will be forced to adapt to these changes and will keep improving to meet these new challenges.

Another fundamental concept that must be followed is that of progression. Progression is increasing the training stress from workout to workout. This can be accomplished by gradually increasing the weight while keeping the sets, reps, and rest periods constant. Another example of progression would be to keep the weight, sets, and reps constant while gradually reducing the rest periods between sets. The beautiful thing about staying consistent with your resistance training program is that progression is a natural byproduct of consistency. If your lifting intensity is consistently high, then it is only a matter of time until you are able to handle heavier loads or do more sets during a given training routine.

Nutrition for Lean Body Mass

Have you been eating 5–6 times a day while making sure to include protein in each meal? If so, you have also been eating in a way that will increase lean body mass. Our nutritional guidelines not only supply you with energy-yielding nutrients and prepare you for optimal performance and health, they also allow you to fully recover from games and practices and are designed for increasing lean body mass.

There is one nutritional area, however, that is a little different when it comes to training for increasing lean body mass and resistance training—the time period before the training session and immediately after the training session. These time periods are referred to as the anabolic window, when accelerated muscle building and recovery takes place. During these two time periods, we recommend that you consume a preworkout beverage and a postworkout beverage containing carbohydrates and protein. Scientific studies have shown that protein synthesis (the building of muscle) is actually accelerated when resistance training is combined with such carbohydrate/protein drinks. However, the anabolic window is limited, so it is imperative that you ingest some type of liquid beverage about thirty minutes before your workout and then immediately after your training session. These two "fluid meals" should be in addition to your other 5–6 meals per day. If this puts you in a state of consuming 300–500 more calories than your maintenance levels, this is acceptable. When trying to gain lean body mass, it is advisable to increase your calories (by approximately 500 calories) above your total daily energy expenditure.

You may be wondering what types of carbohydrates and protein should be consumed during these time periods. In order to answer this question, we need to learn a little bit about the available types of carbohydrates and proteins. Carbohydrates are classified into two categories: low glycemic and high glycemic. While all carbohydrates are converted into glucose (sugar) in the blood, high-glycemic carbohydrates are converted to glucose faster than low-glycemic ones. High-glycemic carbohydrates are often found in fruit juices, sugared drink mixes, and many common sports nutrition drinks. High-glycemic carbohydrates also raise the levels of the hormone insulin, a powerful hormone that causes these high-glycemic carbs to be stored in the muscles as glycogen. Insulin is a very anabolic (muscle building) hormone itself, and it also helps protein do its job of increasing muscle mass.

The type of protein that should be consumed during this anabolic window is one that contains high levels of branched-chain amino acids (BCAAs). Amino acids are the building blocks of proteins, and all proteins are comprised of approximately 20 amino acids. Three of these amino acids—leucine, isoleucine, and valine—are referred to as the branched-chain amino acids. Whey is a very popular protein supplement and contains lots of BCAAs.

So make sure that your pre- and postworkout supplement contains high-glycemic carbohydrates and whey protein (or other protein with plenty of BCAAs). Because high-glycemic carbohydrates induce insulin secretion, by ingesting both high-glycemic carbs and protein, you get a compounded effect—insulin also helps to facilitate the transport of the amino acids into the muscle cells, where they can be utilized to build lean muscle mass. This type of nutritional timing is what will separate you from your competition. Do not just read these nutritional secrets—apply them on a consistent basis.

Appendix A

Sample Weight Training Workouts
HIGH SCHOOL LEVEL

FRESHMEN/SOPHOMORE—EARLY OFF-SEASON (sets x reps)

MONDAY						
	Week 1	**Week 2**	**Week 3**	**Week 4**	**Week 5**	**Week 6–9**
Rotator Cuff Series	1 x 15	1 x 15	1 x 15	1 x 15	1 x 15	2 x 15
Squat	3 x 4	3 x 6	3 x 8	3 x 10	3 x 12	3 x 8
Clean Dead Lift (Frosh)	3 x 5	3 x 5	3 x 5	3 x 5	3 x 5	3 x 5
Clean Pull technique work (Soph.)	5 x 5	5 x 5	5 x 5	5 x 5	5 x 5	5 x 5
Lat Pull Down	3 x 6	3 x 8	3 x 10	3 x 12	3 x 15	3 x 10
Dumbbell Row	3 x 6	3 x 8	3 x 10	3 x 12	3 x 15	3 x 10
Ball Squeeze, 3 x 3	2 sec	3 sec	4 sec	5 sec	6 sec	3 sec
Hammer	1 x 10	1 x 12	1 x 15	2 x 10	2 x 12	2 x 15
Seated Twist	3 x 20	3 x 24	3 x 28	3 x 32	3 x 36	3 x 40

WEDNESDAY						
	Week 1	**Week 2**	**Week 3**	**Week 4**	**Week 5**	**Week 6–9**
Rotator Cuff Series	1 x 15	1 x 15	1 x 15	1 x 15	1 x 15	2 x 15
Clean Dead Lift (Frosh)	3 x 4	3 x 6	3 x 8	3 x 10	3 x 12	3 x 8
Clean Pull technique work (Soph.)	5 x 5	5 x 5	5 x 5	5 x 5	5 x 5	5 x 5
Bench Press	3 x 4	3 x 6	3 x 8	3 x 10	3 x 12	3 x 8
Lat Pull Down	3 x 6	3 x 8	3 x 10	3 x 12	3 x 15	3 x 10

Lying Leg Curl	3 x 8	3 x 10	3 x 12	3 x 15	3 x 20	3 x 15
Hammer	1 x 10	1 x 12	1 x 15	2 x 10	2 x 12	2 x 15
Lying Twist	3 x 20	3 x 24	3 x 28	3 x 32	3 x 36	3 x 40

FRIDAY						
	Week 1	**Week 2**	**Week 3**	**Week 4**	**Week 5**	**Week 6–9**
Rotator Cuff Series	1 x 15	1 x 15	1 x 15	1 x 15	1 x 15	2 x 15
Squat	3 x 4	3 x 6	3 x 8	3 x 10	3 x 12	3 x 8
Bench Press	3 x 4	3 x 6	3 x 8	3 x 10	3 x 12	3 x 8
Dumbbell Row	3 x 6	3 x 8	3 x 10	3 x 12	3 x 15	3 x 10
Lying Leg Curl	3 x 8	3 x 10	3 x 12	3 x 15	3 x 20	3 x 15
Ball Squeeze, 3 x 3	2 sec	3 sec	4 sec	5 sec	6 sec	3 sec
Lying Twist	3 x 20	3 x 24	3 x 28	3 x 32	3 x 36	3 x 40
Seated Twist	3 x 20	3 x 24	3 x 28	3 x 32	3 x 36	3 x 40

Notes: Ascending repetitions (beginning with light weight, progressing from low to high repetition) is used for teaching technique and limiting muscle soreness attributed to high repetition programs for beginners. Sophomores will be learning the Clean Pull and during this technique period little attention is paid to the amount of weight used. It is all about perfecting technique.

FRESHMEN/SOPHOMORE—
LATE OFF-SEASON (sets x reps)

Monday	Rotator Cuff Series	2 x 12
	Squat	5 x 5
	Clean Dead Lift (Frosh)	3 x 5
	Clean Pull technique work (Soph.)	5 x 5
	Lat Pull Down	3 x 8
	Dumbbell Row	3 x 8
	Ball Squeeze, 3 x 6	3 sec
	Hammer	3 x 8
	Seated Twist	3 x 20
Wednesday	Rotator Cuff Series	2 x 12
	Clean Dead Lift (Frosh)	5 x 5
	Clean Pull technique work (Soph.)	5 x 5
	Bench Press	5 x 5

	Lat Pull Down	3 x 8
	Lying Leg Curl	4 x 10
	Hammer	3 x 8
	Seated Twist	3 x 20
	Lying Twist	3 x 40
Friday	Rotator Cuff Series	2 x 12
	Squat	3 x 5
	Bench Press	3 x 5
	Dumbbell Row	3 x 8
	Lying Leg Curl	4 x 10
	Ball Squeeze, 3 x 6	3 sec
	Seated Twist	3 x 20
	Lying Twist	3 x 40

Notes: A decrease in repetitions, but not below five reps. Because the beginning athlete is continually developing physically, there is little scientific reason to change the existing menu by either adding or deleting exercises.

FRESHMEN/SOPHOMORE—PRESEASON (sets x reps)

Monday	Rotator Cuff Series	1 x 15
	Squat	3 x 5
	Clean Dead Lift (Frosh)	3 x 5 (50% of Wednesday weight)
	Clean Pull (Soph.)	60% x 3 x 5
	Dumbbell Row	3 x 5–8
	Hammer	3 x 8
	Lying Twist	3 x 20
Wednesday	Rotator Cuff Series	1 x 15
	Clean Dead Lift (Frosh)	3 x 5
	Clean Pull (Soph.)	60% x 3 x 5
	Bench Press	3 x 5
	Lat Pull Down	3 x 5–8
	Lying Leg Curl	4 x 8–12
	Ball Squeeze, 2 x 3	4 sec
	Seated Twist	3 x 20
	Lying Twist	3 x 40

Friday	Rotator Cuff Series	1 x 15
	Squat	3 x 10 (50% of Monday weight)
	Bench Press	3 x 10 (50% of Wednesday weight)
	Dumbbell Row	3 x 5–8
	Lying Leg Curl	4 x 8–12

Notes: When baseball activity increases, emphasis on weight training decreases and the exercise menu shortens. Post off-season testing allows for the assigning of percentages to the core lifts. On Mondays, performing the clean dead lift before the squat would fatigue the lower back and increase the risk of injury while squatting. Therefore, the squat is performed first and the clean dead lift follows, using 50% of the weight used on the heavier Wednesday workout. Sophomores would have tested for the maximum in the Clean Pull; percentages can now be assigned to the training plan.

FRESHMEN/SOPHOMORE—IN-SEASON (sets x reps)

Monday or Day One	Rotator Cuff Series	1 x 15
	Squat	50% x 3 x 10
	Clean Dead Lift (Frosh)	75% x 3 x 8
	Clean Pull (Soph.)	85% x 3 x 5
	Bench Press	75% x 3 x 8
	Two-Arm Bent Lateral Raise	4 x 8–12
	Lying Leg Curls	5 x 8–12
	Seated Row	4 x 8–12
	Gripper	3 x 10
Wednesday or Day Two	Rotator Cuff Series	1 x 15
	Squat	75% x 3 x 8
	Clean Dead Lift (Frosh)	50% x 3 x 5
	Clean Pull (Soph.)	55% x 3 x 5
	Bench Press	60% x 3 x 10
	Two-Arm Bent Lateral Raise	4 x 8–12
	Lying Leg Curls	5 x 8–12
	Seated Row	4 x 8–12
	Hammer	3 x 10

Notes: High repetitions are usually not appropriate for in-season training, but this level of athlete is still developing and needs the work; an exception might be given to the freshman who is an everyday player or starting pitcher. Workouts are two times per week, based on the weekly game schedule.

JUNIOR/SENIOR—EARLY OFF-SEASON (sets x reps)

MONDAY				
	Week 1	**Week 2**	**Week 3**	**Week 4**
Rotator Cuff Series	1 x 15	1 x 15	1 x 15	1 x 15
Clean Pull	60% x 3 x 8	65% x 3 x 8	70% x 5 x 5	75% x 5 x 5
One-Leg Squat	3 x 10	3 x 10	3 x 8	3 x 8
Two-Arm Dumbbell Lateral Raise	3 x 12	3 x 12	3 x 12	3 x 12
One-Arm Lat Pull Down	3 x 12	3 x 12	3 x 12	3 x 12
Lying Leg Curl	4 x 15	4 x 15	4 x 12	4 x 12
Gripper	2 x 12	2 x 12	2 x 12	2 x 12
Hammer	2 x 15	2 x 15	3 x 10	3 x 10
One-Way Chop, top	2 x 10	2 x 10	2 x 10	2 x 10

WEDNESDAY				
	Week 1	**Week 2**	**Week 3**	**Week 4**
Rotator Cuff Series	1 x 15	1 x 15	1 x 15	1 x 15
Squat	60% x 3 x 8	65% x 3 x 8	70% x 3 x 8	75% x 3 x 8
Bent-Leg Dead Lift with Dumbbells	3 x 10	3 x 10	3 x 8	3 x 8
Bench Press	60% x 3 x 10	65% x 3 x 8	70% x 3 x 8	75% x 3 x 8
Two-Arm Bent Lateral Raise	3 x 12	3 x 12	3 x 12	3 x 12
One-Arm Lat Pull Down	3 x 12	3 x 12	3 x 12	3 x 12
Ball Squeeze, 2 x 6	2 sec	3 sec	4 sec	5 sec
Gripper	2 x 12	2 x 12	2 x 12	2 x 12
Standing Twist	3 x 20	3 x 24	3 x 28	3 x 32
One-Way Chop, top	2 x 10	2 x 10	2 x 10	2 x 10

FRIDAY				
	Week 1	**Week 2**	**Week 3**	**Week 4**
Rotator Cuff Series	1 x 15	1 x 15	1 x 15	1 x 15
Clean Pull	60% x 3 x 5	65% x 3 x 5	70% x 3 x 5	75% x 3 x 5

Bent-Leg Dead Lift with Dumbbells Dead Lift	3 x 5	3 x 5	3 x 5	3 x 5
Bench Press	60% x 3 x 10	60% x 3 x 10	60% x 3 x 10	60% x 3 x 10
Two-Arm Dumbbell Lateral Raise	3 x 12	3 x 12	3 x 12	3 x 12
Two-Arm Bent Lateral Raise	3 x 12	3 x 12	3 x 12	3 x 12
Lying Leg Curl	4 x 15	4 x 15	4 x 12	4 x 12
Ball Squeeze, 2 x 6	2 sec	3 sec	4 sec	5 sec
Hammer	2 x 15	2 x 15	3 x 10	3 x 10
Standing Twist	3 x 20	3 x 24	3 x 28	3 x 32

Notes: After 1–2 years of training, the athlete can begin the year with loads based on percentages of maximum lifts. The increased menu length is for more trained athletes. Trained athletes may not need ascending repetitions. Notice the increased menu length for the older athletes.

JUNIOR/SENIOR—LATE OFF-SEASON (sets x reps)

	MONDAY			
	WEEK 10	**WEEK 11**	**WEEK12**	**WEEK 13**
Rotator Cuff Series	2 x 12	2 x 12	2 x 12	2 x 12
Clean Pull	85% x 3 x 3	80% x 5 x 3	85% x 3 x 5	80% x 5 x 5
One-Leg Squat	4 x 5	4 x 5	4 x 5	4 x 5
Two-Arm Dumbbell Lateral Raise	3 x 6	3 x 6	3 x 6	3 x 6
One-Arm Lat Pull Down	3 x 6	3 x 6	3 x 6	3 x 6
Lying Leg Curl	5 x 8	5 x 8	5 x 8	5 x 8
Gripper	3 x 10	3 x 10	3 x 10	3 x10
Hammer	3 x 8	3 x 8	3 x 8	3 x 8
Three-Way Chop	2 x 10	2 x 10	2 x 10	2 x 10

	WEDNESDAY			
	WEEK 10	**WEEK 11**	**WEEK 12**	**WEEK 13**
Rotator Cuff Series	1 x 15	1 x 15	1 x 15	1 x 15
Squat	85% x 3 x 4	80% x 3 x 4	85% x 3 x 5	80% x 3 x 6
Bench Press	80% x 3 x 4	85% x 4 x 4	90% x 3 x 3	80% x 3 x 5
Two-Arm Bent Lateral Raise	4 x 6	4 x 6	4 x 6	4 x 6
One-Arm Lat Pull Down	4 x 6	4 x 6	4 x 6	4 x 6
Ball Squeeze, 2 x 6	2 sec	3 sec	4 sec	5 sec
Gripper	3 x 10	3 x 10	3 x 10	3 x 10
Standing Twist	3 x 16	3 x 16	3 x 16	3 x 16
Three-Way Chop	2 x 10	2 x 10	2 x 10	2 x 10

	FRIDAY			
	WEEK 10	**WEEK 11**	**WEEK 12**	**WEEK 13**
Rotator Cuff Series	1 x 15	1 x 15	1 x 15	1 x 15
Clean Pull	60% x 5 x 5	65% x 5 x 5	70% x 5 x 5	75% x 5 x 5
Bench Press	60% x 3 x 10	60% x 3 x 8	60% x 3 x 5	60% x 3 x 10
Two-Arm Dumbbell Lateral Raise	3 x 6	3 x 6	3 x 6	3 x 6
Two-Arm Bent Lateral Raise	4 x 6	4 x 6	4 x 6	4 x 6
Lying Leg Curl	5 x 8	5 x 8	5 x 8	5 x 8
Ball Squeeze, 2 x 6	2 sec	3 sec	4 sec	5 sec
Hammer	3 x 8	3 x 8	3 x 8	3 x 8
Standing Twist	3 x 20	3 x 24	3 x 28	3 x 32

Notes: There is repetition reduction in the supplemental exercises. Greater loads are used in the core lifts (80 to 85 percent) than earlier in the cycle. The one-leg squat following heavy clean pulls allows for concentrated leg training without excessive loading of the lower back, considering that fatigue could be a factor following an Olympic movement. Because the load is heavier in the core lifts, it is necessary to lighten the second of the two workouts. For example, on Monday, clean pull 85% x 3 x 3; on Friday, clean pull 60% x 5 x 5.

JUNIOR/SENIOR—PRESEASON (sets x reps)

Monday	Rotator Cuff Series	1 x 15
	Clean Pull	80% x 3 x 3
	One-Leg Squat	3 x 5
	One-Arm Dumbbell Lateral Raise	3 x 6
	Two-Arm Lat Pull Down	4 x 6
	Lying Leg Curl	3 x 8
	Gripper	2 x 10
Wednesday	Rotator Cuff Series	1 x 15
	Squat	85% x 3 x 3
	Bench Press	80% x 3 x 5
	Two-Arm Bent Lateral Raise	4 x 6
	One-Arm Lat Pull Down	4 x 6
	Ball Squeeze, 2 x 3	4 sec
	Standing Twist	2 x 30
Friday	Rotator Cuff Series	1 x 15
	Clean Pull	70% x 3 x 5
	Bench Press	70% x 3 x 5
	Two-Arm Dumbbell Lateral Raise	4 x 6
	Two-Arm Bent Lateral Raise	3 x 6
	Lying Leg Curl	3 x 8
	Hammer	3 x 8
	Standing Twist	2 x 30

JUNIOR/SENIOR—IN-SEASON (sets x reps)

MONDAY			
	WEEK 1	WEEK 2	WEEK 3	WEEK 4
Rotator Cuff Series	1 x 15			
Clean Pull	80% x 3 x 5	65% x 3 x 5	85% x 3 x 5	70% x 3 x 5
Squat	60% x 3 x 5	80% x 3 x 4	60% x 3 x 5	80% x 3 x 4
Bench Press	80% x 3 x 5	85% x 3 x 4	90% x 3 x 2	80% x 3 x 5
Two-Arm Dumbbell Lateral Raise	3 x 5–8	3 x 5–8	3 x 5–8	3 x 5–8
One-Arm Bent Lateral Raise	3 x 5–8	3 x 5–8	3 x 5–8	3 x 5–8
Dumbbell Row	4 x 5–8	4 x 5–8	4 x 5–8	4 _x 5–8
Lying Leg Curls	5 x 8–12	5 x 8–12	5 x 8–12	5 x 8–12
Gripper	3 x 10	3 x 10	3 x 10	3 x 10

WEDNESDAY			
	WEEK 1	WEEK 2	WEEK 3	WEEK 4
Rotator Cuff Series	1 x 15			
Clean Pull	70% x 3 x 5	75% x 3 x 5	70% x 3 x 5	75% x 3 x 5
One-Leg Squat	3 x 5–8	3 x 5–8	3 x 5–8	3 x 5–8
Bench Press	70% x 3 x 5	75% x 3 x 5	70% x 3 x 5	70% x 3 x 5
Two-Arm Dumbbell Lateral Raise	1–3 x 5–8	1–3 x 5–8	1–3 x 5–8	1–3 x 5–8
One-Arm Bent Lateral Raise	1–3 x 5–8	1–3 x 5–8	1–3 x 5–8	1–3 x 5–8
Dumbbell Row	2–4 x 5–8	2–4 x 5–8	2–4 x 5–8	2–4 x 5–8
Lying Leg Curls	2–5 x 8–12	2–5 x 8–12	2–5 x 8–12	2–5 x 8–12
Gripper	1–3 x 10	1–3 x 3 x 10	1–3 x 10	1–3 x 3 x 10

Notes: Traditional medium-low repetitions comprise the in-season program. Notice the week-to-week alternation of heavy squatting and pulling. This enables the athlete and coach to concentrate on one of the two lower body movements per workout, without the other movement suffering in intensity. This also limits the possibility of overtraining the lower body, leading to fatigue or injury.

High School Weight Training Summary

The fundamental themes in comparing and contrasting the workouts are:

1. These are athletes ages 13–18 who need nothing other than the most basic exercises. Physiologically and chronologically, simple programs provide the best short- and long-term results.

2. Weight training sessions longer than 60 minutes are excessive and in some instances provide less development than shorter, intense workouts.

3. Younger athletes need more volume (repetition) for learning technique and preparing for heavier loads in the later years. Preparation should never be cut short or hastened.

4. Aside from the freshman year, the training periods offer illustrations of progressions (heavier weights, more exercises) from year to year and should not be misinterpreted as precise examples.

Appendix B

Sample Weight Training Workouts
COLLEGE LEVEL

FRESHMEN—EARLY OFF-SEASON (sets x reps)

MONDAY				
	WEEK 1	**WEEK 2**	**WEEK 3**	**WEEK 4**
Rotator Cuff Series	2 x 15	2 x 15	2 x 15	2 x 15
Clean Dead Lift	3 x 5	4 x 5	5 x 5	6 x 5
One-Leg Squat	3 x 4	3 x 6	3 x 8	3 x 10
Lying Leg Curls	5 x 6	5 x 8	5 x 10	5 x 12
Two-Arm Dumbbell Lateral Raise	3 x 6	3 x 8	3 x 10	3 x 12
Bent-Leg Dead Lift with Dumbbell	3 x 3	3 x 5	3 x 7	3 x 10
Seated Cable Rows	4 x 6	4 x 8	4 x 10	4 x 12
Two-Arm Lat Pull Down	4 x 6	4 x 8	4 x 10	4 x 12
Dumbbell Shrugs	3 x 6	3 x 8	3 x 10	3 x 12
Triceps Push Down	3 x 6	3 x 8	3 x 10	3 x 12
Deviation	2 x 8	2 x 10	2 x 12	2 x 15
Seated Twists*	3 x 10	3 x 14	3 x 18	3 x 22
Lying Twists*	3 x 10	3 x 14	3 x 18	3 x 22

*Repetitions are more important than the weight being used.

WEDNESDAY

	Week 1	Week 2	Week 3	Week 4
Rotator Cuff Series	2 x 15	2 x 15	2 x 15	2 x 15
Squat	3 x 5	4 x 5	5 x 5	6 x 5
Bench Press	3 x 4	3 x 6	3 x 8	3 x 10
Lying Leg Curls	5 x 6	5 x 8	5 x 10	5 x 12
Two-Arm Bent Lateral Raise	4 x 6	4 x 8	4 x 10	4 x 12
Bent-Leg Dead Lift with Dumbbell	3 x 3	3 x 5	3 x 7	3 x 10
Two-Arm Lat Pull Down	4 x 6	4 x 8	4 x 10	4 x 12
Barbell Curls	3 x 6	3 x 8	3 x 10	3 x 12
Triceps Push Down	3 x 6	3 x 8	3 x 10	3 x 12
Gripper	2 x 8	2 x 10	2 x 12	2 x 15
Lying Twists	3 x 10	3 x 14	3 x 18	3 x 22
Three-Way Chop*	1 x 10	1 x 10	1 x 10	1 x 10

*Repetitions are more important than the weight being used.

FRIDAY

	Week 1	Week 2	Week 3	Week 4
Rotator Cuff Series	2 x 15	2 x 15	2 x 15	2 x 15
Clean Dead Lift	3 x 5	4 x 5	5 x 5	6 x 5
Bench Press	3 x 4	3 x 6	3 x 8	3 x 10
Two-Arm Dumbbell Lateral Raise	3 x 6	3 x 8	3 x 10	3 x 12
Two-Arm Bent Lateral Raise	4 x 6	4 x 8	4 x 10	4 x 12
Seated Cable Rows	4 x 6	4 x 8	4 x 10	4 x 12
Dumbbell Shrugs	3 x 6	3 x 8	3 x 10	3 x 12
Barbell Curls	3 x 6	3 x 8	3 x 10	3 x 12
Deviation	2 x 8	2 x 10	2 x 12	2 x 15
Gripper	2 x 8	2 x 10	2 x 12	2 x 15
Three-Way Chop	1 x 10	1 x 10	1 x 10	1 x 10
Seated Twists	3 x 10	3 x 14	3 x 18	3 x 22

Notes: Ascending repetitions allow the college freshmen to ease into what will probably be a more intensive, consistent weight-training program, as well as a new year-round commitment to baseball activity. Additionally, as a college coach, one cannot assume a background of training; therefore, implementing a basic, beginning program is a safe idea. Deviation and gripper are only two sets each, reducing the chance of forearm fatigue that the freshman athlete might experience with the significant increase of baseball activity at the college level.

FRESHMEN—LATE OFF-SEASON (sets x reps)

Monday	Rotator Cuff Series	2 x 15
	Clean Dead Lift	5 x 3
	One-Leg Squat	3 x 5
	Lying Leg Curls	5 x 8
	Two-Arm Dumbbell Lateral Raise	3 x 8
	Bent-Leg Dead Lift with Dumbbell	3 x 5
	Seated Cable Rows	4 x 8
	Two-Arm Lat Pull Down	4 x 8
	Dumbbell Shrugs	3 x 8
	Triceps Push Down	3 x 8
	Deviation	2 x 8
	Seated Twists	3 x 14 (add weight instead of increasing repetition)
	Lying Twists	3 x 14 (place medicine ball between knees for resistance)
Wednesday	Rotator Cuff Series	2 x 15
	Squat	3 x 5
	Bench Press	3 x 5
	Lying Leg Curls	5 x 8
	Two-Arm Bent Lateral Raise	4 x 8
	Bent-Leg Dead Lift with Dumbbell	3 x 5
	Two-Arm Lat Pull Down	4 x 8
	Barbell Curls	3 x 8
	Triceps Push Down	3 x 8
	Gripper	2 x 8
	Lying Twists	3 x 14 (place medicine ball between knees for resistance)
	Three-Way Chop	2 x 10 (add weight instead of increasing resistance)

Friday	Rotator Cuff Series	2 x 15
	Clean Dead Lift	3 x 5 (50% of Monday weight)
	Bench Press	3 x 5
	Two-Arm Dumbbell Lateral Raise	3 x 8
	Two-Arm Bent Lateral Raise	4 x 8
	Seated Cable Rows	4 x 8
	Dumbbell Shrugs	3 x 8
	Barbell Curls	3 x 8
	Deviation	2 x 8
	Gripper	2 x 8
	Three-Way Chop	2 x 10 (add weight instead of increasing resistance)
	Seated Twists	3 x 14 (add weight instead of increasing resistance)

Notes: Nothing fancy here—a decrease in repetition from the higher-rep, early off-season program; these are midrange repetitions prior to off-season strength testing. Friday's dead lift is lighter than Monday's for three reasons: (1) continued technical work on the movement in preparation for the clean pull, (2) a cautious approach in regard to the lower back during 5–6 days of fall baseball while intensely weight training, and (3) due to heavy squatting on Wednesday, the athlete can reduce the risk of back injury by the use of light weights in the clean dead lift.

FRESHMEN—PRESEASON (sets x reps)

Monday	Rotator Cuff Series	2 x 15
	Clean Dead Lift	70%–85% x 3–5 x 5
	One-Leg Squat	3 x 3
	Lying Leg Curls (1 leg)	5 x 5
	One-Arm Dumbbell Lateral Raise	3 x 5
	Bent-Leg Dead Lift with Dumbbell	3 x 5
	One-Arm Cable Row	4 x 5
	One-Arm Lat Pull Down	4 x 5
	Dumbbell Shrugs	3 x 5
	Triceps Push Down	3 x 5
	Deviation	2 x 8
	Two-Way Chop, top and bottom	1 x 15

Wednesday	Rotator Cuff Series	2 x 15
	Squat	75%–85% x 3 x 3–5
	Bench Press	75%–85% x 3 x 3–5
	Lying Leg Curls	5 x 5
	One-Arm Bent Lateral Raise	4 x 5
	Bent-Leg Dead Lift with Dumbbell	3 x 5
	One-Arm Lat Pull Down	4 x 5
	Barbell Curls	3 x 5
	Triceps Push Down	3 x 5
	Gripper	2 x 8
	Two-Way Chop, top and bottom	1 x 15
	Lying Twist	3 x 10 (place medicine ball between knees for resistance)
Friday	Rotator Cuff Series	2 x 15
	Clean Dead Lift	60%–75% x 3–5 x 3
	Bench Press	60%–75% x 3–5 x 5
	One-Arm Dumbbell Lateral Raise	3 x 5
	One-Arm Bent Lateral Raise	4 x 5
	One-Arm Cable Row	4 x 5
	Dumbbell Shrugs	3 x 5
	Barbell Curls	3 x 5
	Deviation	2 x 8
	Gripper	2 x 8
	Lying Twist	3 x 10 (place medicine ball between knees for resistance)

Notes: Strength testing is performed following the off-season training program, allowing the athlete to use a weight selected as a percentage of his one-repetition maximum for the clean dead lift, bench press, and squat. Supplemental exercise volume is lowered. Some two-arm or two-leg exercises are now unilateral; this is good for changing the stimulus to the muscle and allowing limbs to work independently.

FRESHMEN—IN-SEASON (sets x reps)

MONDAY			
	WEEK 1	**WEEK 2**	**WEEK 3**	**WEEK 4**
Rotator Cuff Series	2 x 15	2 x 15	2 x 15	2 x 15
Clean Dead Lift	70% x 3 x 5	80% x 3 x 5	60% x 3 x 3	85% x 4 x 3
Squat	70% x 3 x 5	65% x 3 x 5	80% x 3 x 4	70% x 3 x 3
Bench Press	80% x 3 x 4	85% x 3 x 3	70% x 3 x 6	75% x 3 x 6
One-Arm Dumbbell Lateral Raise	3 x 5	3 x 5	3 x 5	3 x 5
One-Arm Bent Lateral Raise	4 x 5	4 x 5	4 x 5	4 x 5
Dumbbell Row	4 x 5	4 x 5	4 x 5	4 x 5
Dumbbell Shrugs	3 x 5	3 x 5	3 x 5	3 x 5
Deviation	2 x 8	2 x 8	3 x 5	3 x 5
One-Way Chop, top	3 x 12	3 x 12	3 x 12	3 x 12

WEDNESDAY			
	WEEK 1	**WEEK 2**	**WEEK 3**	**WEEK 4**
Clean Dead Lift	70% x 3 x 5	50% x 3 x 8	60% x 3 x 5	50% x 3 x 8
One-Leg Squat	3 x 5	3 x 5	3 x 5	3 x 5
Bench Press	60% x 3 x 8	60% x 3 x 8	60% x 3 x 8	60% x 3 x 8
One-Arm Dumbbell Lateral Raise	3 x 5	3 x 5	3 x 5	3 x 5
One-Arm Bent Lateral Raise	4 x 5	4 x 5	4 x 5	4 x 5
Dumbbell Row	4 x 5	4 x 5	4 x 5	4 x 5
Dumbbell Shrugs	3 x 5	3 x 5	3 x 5	3 x 5
Gripper	2 x 8	2 x 8	3 x 5	3 x 5
One-Way Chop, bottom	3 x 12	3 x 12	3 x 12	3 x 12

Notes: Monday shows the alternation of a heavy clean dead lift workout followed by a light squat workout (week 2) and vice versa (week 3). Five repetitions allows for a heavy enough weight to strength train, yet not too heavy or repetitious to produce in-season fatigue or soreness. During longer seasons, it would be necessary to program as high as eight repetitions for 4–6 weeks before returning to lower repetitions. Because freshmen will be continually gaining strength, it will be necessary to strength test during the season (caution should be taken with everyday players) and readjust workouts.

SOPHOMORE/JUNIOR—EARLY OFF-SEASON
(sets x reps)

MONDAY			
	WEEK 1	**WEEK 2**	**WEEK 3**	**WEEK 4**
Rotator Cuff Series	2 x 15	2 x 15	2 x 15	2 x 15
Clean Pull technique work	5 x 5	5 x 5	5 x 5	5 x 5
One-Leg Squat	3 x 4	3 x 6	3 x 8	3 x 10
Two-Arm Dumbbell Lateral Raise	3 x 12	3 x 12	3 x 12	3 x 12
One-Arm Lat Pull Down	4 x 12	4 x 12	4 x 12	4 x 12
Leg Curl (2 legs)	4 x 15	4 x 15	4 x 12	4 x 12
Gripper	2 x 12	2 x 12	2 x 12	2 x 12
Deviation	2 x 15	2 x 15	3 x 10	3 x 10
One-Way Chop, top	2 x 10	2 x 10	2 x 10	2 x 10

WEDNESDAY			
	WEEK 1	**WEEK 2**	**WEEK 3**	**WEEK 4**
Rotator Cuff Series	2 x 15	2 x 15	2 x 15	2 x 15
Squat	60% x 3 x 8	65% x 3 x 8	70% x 3 x 8	75% x 3 x 8
Bent-Leg Dead Lift with Barbell	3 x 10	3 x 10	3 x 8	3 x 8
Bench Press	60% x 3 x 10	65% x 3 x 8	70% x 3 x 8	75% x 3 x 8
Two-Arm Bent Lateral Raise	4 x 12	4 x 12	4 x 12	4 x 12
One-Arm Lat Pull Down	4 x 12	4 x 12	4 x 12	4 x 12
One-Arm Cable Row	4 x 12	4 x 12	4 x 12	4 x 12
Ball Squeeze, 2 x 6	2 sec	3 sec	4 sec	5 sec
Gripper	2 x 12	2 x 12	2 x 12	2 x 12
Standing Twist	3 x 20	3 x 24	3 x 28	3 x 32
One-Way Chop, top	2 x 10	2 x 10	2 x 10	2 x 10

FRIDAY			
	WEEK 1	**WEEK 2**	**WEEK 3**	**WEEK 4**
Rotator Cuff Series	2 x 15	2 x 15	2 x 15	2 x 15
Clean Pull technique work	3 x 5	3 x 5	3 x 5	3 x 5
Bent-Leg Dead Lift with Barbell	3 x 10	3 x 10	3 x 8	3 x 8
Bench Press	60% x 3 x 10	60% x 3 x 10	60% x 3 x 10	60% x 3 x 10
Two-Arm Dumbbell Lateral Raise	3 x 12	3 x 12	3 x 12	3 x 12
Two-Arm Bent Lateral Raise	4 x 12	4 x 12	4 x 12	4 x 12
One-Arm Cable Row	4 x 12	4 x 12	4 x 12	4 x 12
Leg Curl (2 legs)	4 x 15	4 x 15	4 x 12	4 x 12
Ball Squeeze, 2 x 6	2 sec	3 sec	4 sec	5 sec
Deviation	2 x 15	2 x 15	3 x 10	3 x 10
Standing Twist	3 x 20	3 x 24	3 x 28	3 x 32

Notes: After one year of training, the athlete begins with high repetitions instead of ascending repetitions in the supplemental lifts. The clean pull will be taught during this time. Careful attention is paid to technique, with virtually no importance is given to poundage; low repetitions allow for learning to occur without the presence of fatigue.

SOPHOMORE/JUNIOR—
LATE OFF-SEASON (sets x reps)

MONDAY				
	Week 8	**Week 9**	**Week 10**	**Week 11**
Rotator Cuff Series	2 x 15	2 x 15	2 x 15	2 x 15
Clean Pull technique work	5 x 5	5 x 5	5 x 5	5 x 5
Clean Pull (if strength tested)	60% x 5 x 5	65% x 5 x 5	70% x 5 x 5	75% x 5 x 5
One-Leg Squat	3 x 5	3 x 5	3 x 5	3 x 5
Two-Arm Dumbbell Lateral Raise	4 x 5	4 x 5	4 x 5	4 x 5
One-Arm Lat Pull Down	5 x 5	5 x 5	5 x 5	5 x 5
Leg Curl (2 legs)	5 x 8	5 x 8	5 x 8	5 x 8
Gripper	3 x 6	3 x 6	3 x 6	3 x 6
Deviation	3 x 6	3 x 6	3 x 6	3 x 6
One-Way Chop, top	2 x 6	2 x 6	2 x 6	2 x 6

WEDNESDAY				
	Week 8	**Week 9**	**Week 10**	**Week 11**
Rotator Cuff Series	2 x 15	2 x 15	2 x 15	2 x 15
Squat	80% x 3 x 5	90% x 3 x 1	80% x 3 x 5	90% x 3 x 2
Bent-Leg Dead Lift with Barbell	3 x 4	3 x 4	3 x 4	3 x 4
Bench Press	75% x 3 x 8	80% x 3 x 5	85% x 3 x 4	90% x 3 x 2
Two-Arm Bent Lateral Raise	5 x 5	5 x 5	5 x 5	5 x 5
One-Arm Lat Pull Down	5 x 5	5 x 5	5 x 5	5 x 5
One-Arm Cable Row	5 x 5	5 x 5	5 x 5	5 x 5
Ball Squeeze, 3 x 6	2 sec	2 sec	2 sec	2 sec
Gripper	3 x 6	3 x 6	3 x 6	3 x 6
Standing Twist*	3 x 20	3 x 20	3 x 20	3 x 20
One-Way Chop, top	2 x 6	2 x 6	2 x 6	2 x 6

*Add weight instead of increasing repetition.

FRIDAY			
	WEEK 8	**WEEK 9**	**WEEK 10**	**WEEK 11**
Rotator Cuff Series	2 x 15	2 x 15	2 x 15	2 x 15
Clean Pull technique work	3 x 5	3 x 5	3 x 5	3 x 5
Clean Pull (if strength tested)	60% x 5 x 5	65% x 5 x 5	70% x 5 x 5	75% x 5 x 5
Bent-Leg Dead Lift with Barbell	3 x 4	3 x 4	3 x 4	3 x 4
Bench Press	75% x 3 x 8	80% x 3 x 5	85% x 3 x 4	90% x 3 x 2
Two-Arm Dumbbell Lateral Raise	4 x 5	4 x 5	4 x 5	4 x 5
Two-Arm Bent Lateral Raise	5 x 5	5 x 5	5 x 5	5 x 5
One-Arm Cable Row	5 x 5	5 x 5	5 x 5	5 x 5
Leg Curl (2 legs)	5 x 8	5 x 8	5 x 8	5 x 8
Ball Squeeze, 3 x 6	2 sec	2 sec	2 sec	2 sec
Deviation	3 x 6	3 x 6	3 x 6	3 x 6
Standing Twist*	3 x 20	3 x 20	3 x 20	3 x 20

*Add weight instead of increasing repetition.

Notes: In some areas, there is more than a 50 percent reduction in repetitions, forcing a significant increase in the weight being used, reducing fatigue, and increasing strength. Emphasis will continue on perfecting the clean pull, unless, after several weeks, technique is proficient enough to test the lift. Sets of five repetitions—the maximum limit for Olympic lifting movements—seems to be the correct number to limit fatigue yet complete a good amount of work. There should be little fear of future shoulder problems while bench pressing heavy weight twice per week. Abdominal training emphasis is now on increasing strength by focusing on increasing the weight being used instead of the repetitions; you cannot expect to increase abdominal and rotational strength if you do not increase the resistance being used.

SOPHOMORE/JUNIOR—PRESEASON (sets x reps)

Monday	Rotator Cuff Series	2 x 15
	Clean Pull	70%–90% x 3–5 x 3–5
	One-Leg Squat	3 x 2-5
	One-Arm Dumbbell Lateral Raise	2–4 x 5
	Two-Arm Lat Pull Down	3–5 x 5
	Leg Curl (1 leg)	3–5 x 5

	Deviation	2 x 6
	One-Way Chop, bottom	2 x 6
Wednesday	Rotator Cuff Series	2 x 15
	Squat	75%–90% x 3 x 1–5
	Bent-Leg Dead Lift with Barbell	1–3 x 4
	Bench Press	75%–90% x 3 x 1–5
	One-Arm Bent Lateral Raise	3–5 x 5
	Two-Arm Lat Pull Down	3–5 x 5
	Dumbbell Row	3–5 x 5
	Ball Squeeze, 2 x 6	4 sec
	Standing Twist	3 x 10 (add weight instead of increasing repetition)
	One-Way Chop, bottom	2 x 6
Friday	Rotator Cuff Series	2 x 15
	Clean Pull	60%–80% x 3 x 3–5
	Bent-Leg Dead Lift with Barbell	1-3 x 4
	Bench Press	70%–80% x 3 x 3–5
	One-Arm Dumbbell Lateral Raise	2–4 x 5
	One-Arm Bent Lateral Raise	3–5 x 5
	Dumbbell Row	3–5 x 5
	Leg Curl (1 leg)	3–5 x 5
	Ball Squeeze, 2 x 6	4 sec
	Deviation	2 x 6
	Standing Twist	3 x 10 (add weight instead of increasing repetition)

Notes: If you think that 90 percent in the core lifts is too high during the preseason, remember that athletes should be at their peak power and strength at this time of year, and this does not occur with light weights. Volume is low while lifting heavy in order to limit fatigue and soreness (which typically come from volume, not load). Since baseball activity has increased in intensity and emphasis, it might be necessary to adjust the number of sets performed, which is why we list ranges for sets (i.e., 2–4 x 5) but not repetitions. There is no change in repetitions because increasing repetitions when sets are decreased defeats the purpose of (a) strength training and (b) lowering the number of sets to decrease load and fatigue.

SOPHOMORE/JUNIOR—IN-SEASON (sets x reps)

MONDAY			
	WEEK 1	**WEEK 2**	**WEEK 3**	**WEEK 4**
Rotator Cuff Series	2 x 15	2 x 15	2 x 15	2 x 15
Clean Pull	80% x 5 x 3	90% x 4 x 1	60% x 2 x 5	85% x 5 x 3
Squat	80% x 3 x 3	65% x 3 x 5	90% x 2 x 1	60% x 3 x 3
Bench Press	80% x 3 x 4	85% x 3 x 3	70% x 3 x 6	90% x 2 x 1
One-Arm Dumbbell Lateral Raise	3 x 8	3 x 8	3 x 5	3 x 5
One-Arm Bent Lateral Raise	4 x 8	4 x 8	4 x 5	4 x 5
Dumbbell Row	4 x 8	4 x 8	4 x 5	4 x 5
Leg Curl (1 leg)	4 x 8	4 x 8	4 x 5	4 x 5
Deviation	2 x 8	2 x 8	3 x 5	3 x 5
Two-Way Chop, top and bottom	2 x 10	2 x 10	2 x 10	2 x 10

WEDNESDAY			
	WEEK 1	**WEEK 2**	**WEEK 3**	**WEEK 4**
Rotator Cuff Series	2 x 15	2 x 15	2 x 15	2 x 15
Clean Pull	80% x 3 x 3	70% x 2 x 5	70% x 3 x 5	75% x 3 x 3
One-Leg Squat	3 x 5	3 x 5	3 x 5	3 x 5
Bench Press	80% x 3 x 2	75% x 3 x 4	70% x 3 x 3	70% x 2 x 3
Two-Arm Dumbbell Lateral Raise	1-3 x 8	1-3 x 8	1-3 x 5	1-3 x 5
Two-Arm Bent Lateral Raise	2-4 x 8	2-4 x 8	2-4 x 5	2-4 x 5
Dumbbell Row	2-4 x 8	2-4 x 8	2-4 x 5	2-4 x 5
Leg Curl (2 legs)	2-4 x 8	2-4 x 8	2-4 x 5	2-4 x 5
Ball Squeeze, 2 x 4	6 sec	6 sec	6 sec	6 sec
Lying Twist	2 x 14	2 x 14	2 x 14	2 x 14

Notes: The clean pull and squat will alternate week to week in emphasis; both lifts heavy on the same day is not recommended, especially during the season. Heavy loads (80%–90%) must be used periodically in the beginning of the week during the season if the athlete is to retain as much strength as possible. A second-year or third-year athlete will be able to handle heavier loads than a beginning athlete. Wednesday's core lifts are reduced in intensity (amount of weight lifted) and volume (repetitions) to prepare for the weekend games; it is possible for the supplemental lifts to have the same sets and repetitions on both days early in the season, but they must also be reduced as the season continues. Slight modifications of the same exercise from Monday to Wednesday (one arm to two arms, etc.) will help keep strength levels elevated.

JUNIOR/SENIOR—EARLY OFF-SEASON (sets x reps)

MONDAY			
	WEEK 1	**WEEK 2**	**WEEK 3**	**WEEK 4**
Rotator Cuff Series	2 x 15	2 x 15	2 x 15	2 x 15
Clean Pull	75% x 3 x 5	80% x 3 x 5	75% x 5 x 5	80% x 5 x 5
One-Leg Squat	3 x 4	3 x 6	3 x 8	3 x 10
Two-Arm Dumbbell Lateral Raise	3 x 8	3 x 8	3 x 8	3 x 8
Two-Arm Lat Pull Down	4 x 8	4 x 8	4 x 8	4 x 8
Seated Cable Row	4 x 8	4 x 8	4 x 8	4 x 8
Dumbbell Shrug	3 x 8	3 x 8	3 x 8	3 x 8
Leg Curl (2 legs)	4 x 8	4 x 8	4 x 8	4 x 8
Gripper	2 x 12	2 x 12	2 x 8	2 x 8
Deviation	2 x 15	2 x 15	3 x 10	3 x 10
Three-Way Chop	1 x 10	1 x 10	1 x 10	1 x 10

WEDNESDAY			
	WEEK 1	**WEEK 2**	**WEEK 3**	**WEEK 4**
Rotator Cuff Series	2 x 15	2 x 15	2 x 15	2 x 15
Squat	75% x 4 x 5	80% x 3 x 5	70% x 5 x 5	85% x 4 x 4
Bent-Leg Dead Lift with Barbell	3 x 10	3 x 10	3 x 8	3 x 8
Bench Press	65% x 3 x 8	70% x 3 x 8	75% x 3 x 8	80% x 3 x 6
Incline Dumbbell Bench Press	3 x 8	3 x 8	3 x 8	3 x 8
Two-Arm Bent Lateral Raise	4 x 8	4 x 8	4 x 8	4 x 8
Two-Arm Lat Pull Down	4 x 8	4 x 8	4 x 8	4 x 8

Ball Squeeze, 2 x 6	2 sec	3 sec	4 sec	5 sec
Gripper	2 x 12	2 x 12	2 x 8	2 x 8
Seated Twist	3 x 20	3 x 24	3 x 28	3 x 32
Three-Way Chop	1 x 10	1 x 10	1 x 10	1 x 10

FRIDAY				
	WEEK 1	**WEEK 2**	**WEEK 3**	**WEEK 4**
Rotator Cuff Series	2 x 15	2 x 15	2 x 15	2 x 15
Clean Pull	70% x 3 x 5	75% x 3 x 5	70% x 3 x 5	75% x 3 x 5
Bent-Leg Dead Lift with Barbell	3 x 10	3 x 10	3 x 8	3 x 8
Bench Press	60% x 3 x 10	60% x 3 x 10	60% x 3 x 10	60% x 3 x 10
Incline Dumbbell Bench Press	3 x 8	3 x 8	3 x 8	3 x 8
Two-Arm Dumbbell Lateral Raise	3 x 8	3 x 8	3 x 8	3 x 8
Two-Arm Bent Lateral Raise	4 x 8	4 x 8	4 x 8	4 x 8
Seated Cable Row	4 x 8	4 x 8	4 x 8	4 x 8
Dumbbell Shrug	3 x 8	3 x 8	3 x 8	3 x 8
Leg Curl (2 legs)	4 x 8	4 x 8	4 x 8	4 x 8
Ball Squeeze, 2 x 6	2 sec	3 sec	4 sec	5 sec
Deviation	2 x 15	2 x 15	3 x 10	3 x 10
Seated Twist	3 x 20	3 x 24	3 x 28	3 x 32

Notes: This program is typical of the senior athlete and the developed junior. The moderate intensity and high volume clean pull is necessary to begin the year and retrain. After 2–3 years of high repetitions in the early off-season, medium repetitions are suitable because there is no longer a need to build a training base. Following an intense week-2 squat workout, squatting light in week 3 allows the athlete to recover and prepare for a heavy week 4. The Friday bench press workout is lighter than the Wednesday workout to help the stronger, experienced lifter recover. All back-of-the-shoulder and pulling work has additional sets to emphasize balance in the throwing decelerators.

JUNIOR/SENIOR—LATE OFF-SEASON (sets x reps)

MONDAY			
	WEEK 10	**WEEK 11**	**WEEK 12**	**WEEK 13**
Rotator Cuff Series	2 x 15	2 x 15	2 x 15	2 x 15
Clean Pull	85% x 5 x 3	80% x 5 x 5	90% x 5 x 2	95% x 4 x 1
One-Leg Squat	4 x 3	4 x 3	4 x 3	4 x 3
Two-Arm Dumbbell Lateral Raise	3 x 5	3 x 5	3 x 5	3 x 5
Two-Arm Lat Pull Down	5 x 5	5 x 5	5 x 5	5 x 5
Seated Cable Row	5 x 5	5 x 5	5 x 5	5 x 5
Dumbbell Shrug	3 x 5	3 x 5	3 x 5	3 x 5
Leg Curl (2 legs)	5 x 5	5 x 5	5 x 5	5 x 5
Gripper	2 x 6	2 x 6	2 x 6	2 x 6
Deviation	3 x 5	3 x 5	3 x 5	3 x 5
Three-Way Chop	2 x 10	2 x 10	2 x 10	2 x 10

WEDNESDAY			
	WEEK 10	**WEEK 11**	**WEEK 12**	**WEEK 13**
Rotator Cuff Series	2 x 15	2 x 15	2 x 15	2 x 15
Squat	85% x 4 x 4	90% x 3 x 2	80% x 3 x 3	95% x 1
Bent-Leg Dead Lift with Barbell	2 x 5	2 x 5	2 x 5	2 x 5
Bench Press	90% x 3 x 1	80% x 3 x 5	95% x 1	90% x 3 x 2
Incline Dumbbell Bench Press	3 x 5	3 x 5	3 x 5	3 x 5
Two-Arm Bent Lateral Raise	4 x 5	4 x 5	4 x 5	4 x 5
One-Arm Lat Pull Down	4 x 8	4 x 8	4 x 8	4 x 8
Ball Squeeze, 2 x 3	2 sec	3 sec	4 sec	5 sec
Gripper	2 x 6	2 x 6	2 x 6	2 x 6
Seated Twist	3 x 20	3 x 20	3 x 20	3 x 20
Three-Way Chop	1 x 6	1 x 6	1 x 6	1 x 6

	FRIDAY			
	WEEK 10	**WEEK 11**	**WEEK 12**	**WEEK 13**
Rotator Cuff Series	2 x 15	2 x 15	2 x 15	2 x 15
Clean Pull	70% x 2 x 5	75% x 2 x 5	70% x 2 x 5	70% x 2 x 5
Dumbbell Bent Leg Dead Lift	2 x 5	2 x 5	2 x 5	2 x 5
Bench Press	60% x 3 x 5	60% x 3 x 10	60% x 3 x 5	60% x 3 x 5
Incline Dumbbell Bench Press	3 x 5	3 x 5	3 x 5	3 x 5
One-Arm Dumbbell Lateral Raise	3 x 8	3 x 8	3 x 8	3 x 8
One-Arm Bent Lateral Raise	4 x 8	4 x 8	4 x 8	4 x 8
One-Arm Cable Row	4 x 8	4 x 8	4 x 8	4 x 8
Dumbbell Shrug	3 x 5	3 x 5	3 x 5	3 x 5
Leg Curl (1 leg)	4 x 8	4 x 8	4 x 8	4 x 8
Ball Squeeze, 2 x 3	2 sec	3 sec	4 sec	5 sec
Deviation	3 x 5	3 x 5	3 x 5	3 x 5
Seated Twist	3 x 20	3 x 20	3 x 20	3 x 20

Notes: This period has the heaviest clean pull program—the athlete has been trained for this. One-leg squats should be attempted with the heaviest weight possible. Supplemental exercises are low repetition and with the heaviest weight possible. This phase has the heaviest lower-back load (clean pull, squat, one-leg squat) and, as a result, the bent-leg dead lift is a two-set exercise. Creativity to vary stimulus to the muscles is necessary for experienced lifters: use the same exercise with different repetitions and technique, as in the two-arm dumbbell lateral raise on Monday and the one-arm dumbbell lateral raise on Friday.

JUNIOR/SENIOR—PRESEASON (sets x reps)

Monday	Rotator Cuff Series	2 x 15
	Clean Pull	75%–90% x 3–5 x 3
	One-Leg Squat	2–4 x 3–5
	One-Arm Dumbbell Lateral Raise	2–3 x 5
	One-Arm Lat Pull Down	3–5 x 5
	Dumbbell Row	3–5 x 5
	Leg Curl (1 leg)	3–5 x 5
	Gripper	2 x 6
	Deviation	1–3 x 5
	One-Way Chop, middle	2 x 10
Wednesday	Rotator Cuff Series	2 x 15
	Squat	80%–90% x 1–3 x 1–3
	Bench Press	80%–90% x 1–3 x 1–4
	Incline Dumbbell Bench Press	3 x 5
	One-Arm Bent Lateral Raise	3–5 x 5
	One-Arm Lat Pull Down	1–3 x 5
	Ball Squeeze, 1 x 3	4 sec
	Gripper	2 x 6
	Seated Twist	3 x 20
	One-Way Chop, middle	2 x 10
Friday	Rotator Cuff Series	2 x 15
	Clean Pull	60%–70% x 3 x 5
	Bench Press	60%–75% x 3 x 3–5
	Incline Dumbbell Bench Press	1–3 x 5
	One-Arm Dumbbell Lateral Raise	1–3 x 5
	One-Arm Bent Lateral Raise	1–3 x 5
	One-Arm Cable Row	1–3 x 5
	Leg Curl (1 leg)	1–3 x 5
	Ball Squeeze, 2 x 3	2 sec
	Deviation	1–3 x 5
	Seated Twist	3 x 20

Notes: Core lift loads are slightly heavier than for the younger lifters, yet the volumes remain low (squat and clean pull at 90% x 1 x 1 and 90% x 3 x 3, respectively). There is a significant reduction in the supplemental lifts, especially on Wednesday, because the experienced, usually stronger athlete will need more recovery, leading to fewer sets and repetitions. The coach can choose to increase the intensity (heaviest weight possible for more or fewer sets) or decrease the intensity (lighter than normal weight for more or fewer sets).

JUNIOR/SENIOR—IN-SEASON (sets x reps)

MONDAY				
	WEEK 1	WEEK 2	WEEK 3	WEEK 4
Rotator Cuff Series	2 x 15	2 x 15	2 x 15	2 x 15
Clean Pull	80% x 5 x 3	90% x 3 x 2	70% x 2 x 5	85% x 3 x 3
Squat	80% x 3 x 3	65% x 2 x 5	90% x 1 x 3	70% x 2 x 5
Bench Press	80% x 3 x 4	85% x 3 x 3	70% x 3 x 6	90% x 2 x 1
One-Arm Dumbbell Lateral Raise	3 x 8	3 x 8	3 x 5	3 x 5
Two-Arm Bent Lateral Raise	4 x 8	4 x 8	4 x 5	4 x 5
One-Arm Cable Row	4 x 8	4 x 8	4 x 5	4 x 5
Leg Curl (2 leg)	4 x 8	4 x 8	4 x 5	4 x 5
Deviation	1 x 8, 1 x 5	1 x 8, 1 x 5	2 x 6	2 x 6
Two-Way Chop, top and bottom	2 x 10	2 x 10	2 x 10	2 x 10

WEDNESDAY				
	WEEK 1	WEEK 2	WEEK 3	WEEK 4
Rotator Cuff Series	2 x 15	2 x 15	2 x 15	2 x 15
Clean Pull	80% x 3 x 3	70% x 2 x 5	70% x 3 x 5	75% x 3 x 3
One-Leg Squat	3 x 5	3 x 5	3 x 5	3 x 5
Incline Dumbbell Bench Press	3 x 8	3 x 8	3 x 5	3 x 5
Two-Arm Dumbbell Lateral Raise	1–3 x 8	1–3 x 8	1–3 x 5	1–3 x 5
One-Arm Bent Lateral Raise (with cable)	2–4 x 8	2–4 x 8	2–4 x 5	2–4 x 5

Dumbbell Row	2–4 x 8	2–4 x 8	2–4 x 5	2–4 x 5
Leg Curl (1 leg)	2–4 x 8	2–4 x 8	2–4 x 5	2–4 x 5
Gripper	1 x 8, 1 x 5	1 x 8, 1 x 5	2 x 6	2 x 6
Lying Twist	3 x 14	3 x 14	2 x 20	2 x 20

Notes: This is a slightly heavier load in the core lifts for the older athlete. The Wednesday incline dumbbell bench press is a great alternative following an in-season Monday bench press. Supplemental lifts can be altered from Monday to Wednesday by modifying the same exercise (two-arm to one-arm dumbbell lateral raise) or changing the apparatus (cable row to dumbbell row); variety is important for the more trained athlete. Monday illustrates what could be at least a 50% reduction in volume leading into the weekend's games: 1 x 8, 1 x 5 (perform a set of eight repetitions, then increase the resistance and perform five repetitions). Remember, this level of athlete is close to his or her maximum potential, so performing one set of three repetitions at 90% in the squat satisfies the need for intensity without multiple sets.

JUNIOR/SENIOR—LATE IN-SEASON (sets x reps)

MONDAY			
	WEEK 11	**WEEK 12**	**WEEK 13**	**WEEK 14**
---	---	---	---	---
Clean Pull	80% x 3 x 5	90% x 3, 60% x 2 x 5	85% x 3, 80% x 2 x 3	75% x 2 x 5
One-Leg Squat	3 x 5	3 x 5	4 x 2	4 x 2

WEDNESDAY			
	WEEK 11	**WEEK 12**	**WEEK 13**	**WEEK 14**
---	---	---	---	---
Clean Pull	70% x 2 x 5	70% x 2 x 5	75% x 2 x 5	75% x 3 x 3
Squat	80% x 2 x 2	65% x 3 x 5	85% x 1 x 3	60% x 2 x 5

Notes: The more advanced athlete is going to depend on variety as a means to continually improve in strength and power. This variety has already been shown in many of the workouts. For example, in the clean pull you can vary the load in one workout, performing a heavy set followed by a lighter set, to create more power (speed of movement). This technique is analogous to swinging a weighted bat followed by a lighter bat. Also, because the clean pull and squat are maximally loading the lower back, switching the one-leg squat to Monday during mid- to late in-season and making it the "heavy leg day" will unload the back without compromising leg strength. *This can only be done if the heaviest load possible is used in the one-leg squat.* On Wednesday, the squat can be performed with light to medium weights to maintain flexibility in the two-legged movement.

COLLEGE WEIGHT TRAINING SUMMARY

We incorporate subtle but important changes as the athlete becomes more experienced; experienced meaning considerably stronger and technically more advanced in the execution of weight training movements.

1. The senior and advanced junior athlete should be at their peak strength and power. So the need to "push" that athlete with heavier loads *and* repetition is unnecessary. Heavier loads should be the emphasis with very little change in repetitions, especially in the core lifts.

2. As a college coach, despite what the incoming athlete might tell you, treat them as if they are beginning weight trainers. A truly advanced athlete will be evident in a short, necessary time.

3. The college freshman starts with ascending repetitions to gradually adjust to the increased activity and intensity of college baseball as well as to the rigors of college academics.

4. Variety in the supplemental lifts (sets, repetitions, exercise modifications, technique modifications) is a necessary tool in developing the college athlete.

5. Core leg workouts should consist of a squat day and a one-leg squat day. The one-leg squat develops single-leg strength and stability while lessening the stress to the lower back. Strenuous clean pull workouts and heavy squatting, not to mention throwing and swinging nearly every day, makes squatting twice per week a risky proposition for lower-back health.

6. Many baseball injuries are a result of a lack of strength due to programs that recommend light weights and medium to high repetitions. Intense weight training (heaviest possible loads for low repetition zones) promotes strength and teaches the body what all-out effort is, thereby minimizing easily preventable injuries.

Appendix C

Sample Weight Training Workouts PROFESSIONAL LEVEL

OFF-SEASON

Several factors need to be considered when designing and implementing a professional level weight training program:

- Age: less than 18 to 40 years old or more

- Weight training experience in years: 0–20

- Weight training objective: increase muscle mass, maintain flexibility, injury prevention, etc.

- Injury or surgical history: past, present, and future; a history of recurring injury or a trend of treatments (icing, massage, heat therapy, etc.) may indicate the likelihood of a future injury

- Limitation: as a result of injury, surgery, or anatomy

- Risk: a player unable to perform as a result of a weight lifting injury or poor program design impacts an organization, team, players, and coaches more than at any other level

It is the above factors that lead to the many professional baseball programs that have been used. And because of those factors, it makes little sense to criticize or evaluate a program without knowing the underlying variables of an organization's philosophy and processes. Professional baseball is much different than any other level; weight training programs are influenced by more than the physical objectives of programming.

With several objectives to consider, the number of training programs is endless. Because of this, descriptions such as 50%–100% or 3–5 x 4–12 must be used to illustrate the range of program design that a player might encounter.

THREE-DAY SCHEDULE (sets x reps)

MONDAY • *Total body power (clean dead lift, clean pull), quadriceps (squats or one-leg squats), shoulders, trapezius, arms (biceps, triceps), and abdominals/rotational exercises.*

Rotator Cuff Series	1–2 x 10–15
Clean Dead Lift	50%–100% x 1–5 x 1–5
One-Leg Squats	2–5 x 3–10
Two-Arm Dumbbell Lateral Raise	2–3 x 4–12
Two-Arm Bent Lateral Raise	3–5 x 4–12
Dumbbell Shrugs	2–3 x 4–12
Dumbbell Curls	2–3 x 4–12
Triceps Push Down	2–4 x 4–12
Lying Twist	2–3 x 10–30
Seated Twist	2–3 x 10–30

WEDNESDAY • *Total body power (clean dead lift, clean pull), chest, hamstrings/lower back, latissimus/rhomboids, arms (biceps, triceps), forearms/grip, abdominals/rotational exercises.*

Rotator Cuff Series	1–2 x 10–15
Clean Dead Lift	50%–80% x 1–3 x 1–5
Dumbbell Flat Bench Press	3–5 x 4–12
Dumbbell Incline Press	3–5 x 4–12
Leg Curls (2 legs)	3–5 x 4–12
Bent-Leg Dead Lift with Dumbbell	2–4 x 4–12
Dumbbell Row	3–5 x 4–12
Two-Arm Lat Pull Down	3–5 x 4–12
Dumbbell Curls	2–3 x 4–12

Triceps Push Down	2–4 x 4–12
Deviation	2–4 x 4–12
Gripper	2–4 x 4–12
Three-Way Chop	1–3 x 10–20

FRIDAY • *Quadriceps (squats or one-leg squats), chest, hamstrings/lower back, shoulders, latissimus/rhomboids, trapezius, forearms/grip, abdominals/rotational exercises.*

Rotator Cuff Series	1–2 x 10–15
Squat	50%–100% x 1–5 x 1–5
Bench Press	50%–100% x 1–5 x 1–5
Incline Barbell Press	50%–100% x 1–5 x 1–5
Leg Curls (2 legs)	3–5 x 4–12
Bent-Leg Dead Lift with Dumbbell	2–4 x 4–12
Two-Arm Dumbbell Lateral Raise	2–3 x 4–12
Two-Arm Bent Lateral Raise	3–5 x 4–12
Seated Cable Row	3–5 x 4–12
Two-Arm Lat Pull Down	3–5 x 4–12
Dumbbell Shrugs	2–3 x 4–12
Deviation	2–4 x 4–12
Gripper	2–4 x 4–12
Lying Twist	2–3 x 10–30
Seated Twist	2–3 x 10–30

FOUR-DAY SCHEDULE (sets x reps)

MONDAY • *Total body power (clean dead lift, clean pull), hamstrings/lower back, latissimus/rhomboids, biceps, and forearms/grip exercises.*

Rotator Cuff Series	1–2 x 10–15
Clean Pull	60%–100% x 1–5 x 1–5
Leg Curls (1 leg)	3–5 x 4–12
Bent-Leg Dead Lift with Dumbbell	2–4 x 4–12
Seated Cable Row	3–5 x 4–12
Two-Arm Lat Pull Down	3–5 x 4–12

Barbell Curls	2–3 x 4–12
Deviation	2–4 x 4–12
Gripper	2–4 x 4–12

TUESDAY • *Quadriceps (squats or one-leg squats), chest, shoulders/trapezius, triceps, abdominals/rotational exercises.*

Rotator Cuff Series	1–2 x 10–15
Squat	50%–100% x 1–5 x 1–5
Flat Dumbbell Bench Press	3–5 x 4–12
Incline Barbell Bench Press	50%–100% x 1–5 x 1–5
One-Arm Dumbbell Lateral Raise	2–3 x 4–12
One-Arm Bent Lateral Raise with Cable	3–5 x 4–12
Dumbbell Shrugs	2–3 x 4–12
Triceps Push Down	3–4 x 4–12
Standing Twist	2–3 x 10–30
Lying Twist	2–3 x 10–30

WEDNESDAY • *Off.*

THURSDAY • *Total body power (clean dead lift, clean pull), hamstrings/lower back, latissimus/rhomboids, shoulders/trapezius, biceps, forearms/grip exercises.*

Rotator Cuff Series	1–2 x 10–15
Clean Pull	60%–100% x 1–5 x 1–5
Leg Curls (2 legs)	3–5 x 4–12
Bent-Leg Dead Lift with Barbell	2–4 x 4–12
Dumbbell Row	3–5 x 4–12
One-Arm Lat Pull Down	3–5 x 4–12
Alternate Dumbbell Curls	2–3 x 4–12
Deviation	2–4 x 4–12
Gripper	2–4 x 4–12

FRIDAY • *Quadriceps (squats or one-leg squats), chest, triceps, abdominals/rotational exercises.*

| Rotator Cuff Series | 1–2 x 10–15 |
| One-Leg Squat | 2–5 x 3–10 |

Bench Press	50%–100% x 1–5 x 1–5
Incline Dumbbell Bench Press	3–5 x 4–12
One-Arm Dumbbell Lateral Raise	2–3 x 4–12
One-Arm Bent Lateral Raise with Cable	3–5 x 4–12
Dumbbell Shrugs	2–3 x 4–12
Triceps Push Down	3–4 x 4–12
Standing Twist	2–3 x 10–30
Lying Twist	2–3 x 10–30

FIVE-DAY SCHEDULE (sets x reps)

MONDAY • *Total body power (clean dead lift, clean pull), hamstrings/lower back forearms/grip exercises.*

Clean Pull	60%–100% x 1–5 x 1–5
Leg Curls (1 leg)	3–5 x 4–12
Bent-Leg Dead Lift with Dumbbell	2–4 x 4–12
Deviation	2–4 x 4–12
Gripper	2–4 x 4–12

TUESDAY • *Chest, abdominals/rotational exercises.*

Bench Press	50%–100% x 1–5 x 1–5
Incline Barbell Bench Press	50%–100% x 1–5 x 1–5
Three-Way Chop	1–3 x 10–30
Lying Twist	2–3 x 10–30

WEDNESDAY • *Shoulders/trapezius, forearms/grip exercises.*

Two-Arm Dumbbell Lateral Raise	2–3 x 4–12
One-Arm Bent Lateral Raise with Cable	3–5 x 4–12
Dumbbell Shrugs	2–3 x 4–12
Triceps Push Down	3–4 x 4–12
Deviation	2–4 x 4–12
Gripper	2–4 x 4–12

THURSDAY • *Latissimus/rhomboids exercises.*

Dumbbell Row	3–5 x 4–12
One-Arm Lat Pull Down	3–5 x 4–12
Seated Row	3–5 x 4–12
Barbell Curl	2–3 x 4–12

FRIDAY • *Quadriceps, abdominals/rotational exercises.*

Squat	50%–100% x 1–5 x 1–5
One-Leg Squat	2–5 x 3–10
Three-Way Chop	1–3 x 10–30
Lying Twist	2–3 x 10–30

Bench press and incline barbell bench press: Because this exercise will have the athlete handling the heaviest weight in a shoulder-related movement, particular emphasis is placed on grip and range of motion, which influence the stress to the area. A training range of 50%–100% and 1–5 x 1–5 indicates that the athlete could be using this exercise for any one of several reasons—to maintain flexibility (50%–70%), strength training (80%–100%), lighter sets first building to maximum poundage later in the workout (pyramiding), or building to maximum poundage week to week over the course of the off-season (beginning in week 1 with 50% and the final week at 100%). However, with the repetition range between one and five, there is no emphasis on building muscle, which could lead to changes in the throwing motion and most likely to injury.

Clean dead lift and clean pull: These are seldom-used movements due to (a) overusing the lower back, which is affected by daily fielding, throwing, and swinging; (b) very little expert supervision; and (c) lack of facility. Those who find these lifts of value might use them for the total-body work these lifts provide. The repetition range should be low to enforce technique and in the clean pull to promote speed of movement (power enhancement).

Squat: Another movement that puts the lower back at risk in any population, the squat is a more common lift yet not normally used with maximum poundage. One of the most effective trunk strengtheners (the core), it is performed with a wide range of intensities, showing that the squat can be used to build lower body strength, increase or maintain flexibility, or promote total body effort.

One-leg squat: Developing single-leg strength, stability, and flexibility, the professional player might need to retrain this lift by beginning with ascending repetitions after the long season. There are a few ways this exercise can be utilized in this program: emphasis on medium to low repetitions with maximum weight for pure strength; medium to low repetitions with medium to light weight because the squat and the pulls from the ground are of greater importance or to maintain/increase flexibility; or due to back injury or limitation, the squat is performed with light weight and the one-leg squat becomes the primary leg exercise.

Supplemental Lifts: Only first-time lifters or those returning to a full lifting schedule need ascending repetitions at the beginning of the off-season. The wide range of sets and repetitions leads to a wide range of training concepts:

Example: 3–5 x 4–12

- Monday and Wednesday. Both days at maximum poundage, beginning with 3–5 x 12 in week 1 and ending the off-season with 3–5 x 4. These are classical descending repetitions.

- Monday and Wednesday. Both days at maximum poundage, beginning with 3–5 x 4 in week 1 and ending the off-season with 3–5 x 12. These are ascending repetitions, but it emphasizes endurance because it is performed over a longer period and not just in the beginning of the off-season.

  ○ Monday—3–5 x 4–12 with maximum poundage; Wednesday (recovery)—3–5 x 4–12 with 50%–70% of Monday's poundage. The reduction of weight on Wednesday serves as a day of recovery from the more intense Monday, yet not full rest.

  ○ Monday—5 x 8 @ 100 pounds; Wednesday—3 x 8 @ 100 pounds. This is a recovery workout due to fewer sets on Wednesday. In this case, 16 fewer repetitions than Monday at 100 pounds.

○ Monday—3–5 x 4 with maximum poundage; Wednesday—3–5 x 12 with maximum poundage. This training scheme works both muscular strength (Monday) and endurance (Wednesday). However, due to the use of maximum poundage on both days, this type of training is not preferred for prolonged periods because of the chance for overtraining and possible injury. Definitely an advanced technique.

PRESEASON/SPRING TRAINING

The intensity (percentages and weight being used), repetitions, and sets are the same for each exercise, whether the program is a three-day, four-day, or five-day schedule. All the aforementioned programs are beneficial; however, we will illustrate the three-day schedule only.

THREE-DAY SCHEDULE (sets x reps)

DAY ONE • *Total body power (clean dead lift, clean pull), quadriceps (squats or one-leg squats), shoulders, trapezius, arms (biceps, triceps), abdominals/rotational exercises.*

Rotator Cuff Series	1–2 x 10–15
Clean Dead Lift	50%–85% x 1–3 x 1–5
One-Leg Squats	2–3 x 3–5
Two-Arm Dumbbell Lateral Raise	1–3 x 4–6
Two-Arm Bent Lateral Raise	2–4 x 4–6
Dumbbell Shrugs	1–3 x 4–6
Dumbbell Curls	1–3 x 4–6
Triceps Push Down	2–3 x 4–6
Lying Twist	1–3 x 10–20
Seated Twist	1–3 x 10–20

DAY TWO • *Total body power (clean dead lift, clean pull), chest, hamstrings/lower back, latissimus/rhomboids, arms (biceps, triceps), forearms/grip, abdominals/ rotational exercises.*

Rotator Cuff Series	1–2 x 10–15
Clean Dead Lift	50%–85% x 1–3 x 1–5
Flat Dumbbell Bench Press	2–4 x 4–6
Incline Dumbbell Bench Press	2–4 x 4–6
Leg Curls (2 legs)	2–4 x 4–6
Bent-Leg Dead Lift with Dumbbell	1–3 x 4–6
Dumbbell Row	2–4 x 4–6
Two-Arm Lat Pull Down	2–4 x 4–6
Dumbbell Curls	1–3 x 4–6
Triceps Push Down	2–3 x 4–6
Deviation	1–3 x 6–8
Gripper	1–3 x 6–8
Three-Way Chop	1–2 x 8–12

DAY THREE • *Quadriceps (squats or one-leg squats), chest, hamstrings/lower back, shoulders, latissimus/rhomboids, trapezius, forearms/grip, abdominals/rotational exercises.*

Rotator Cuff Series	1–2 x 10–15
Squat	50%–85% x_ 1–3 x 1–5
Bench Press	50%–85% x 1–3 x 1–5
Incline Barbell Bench Press	50%–100% x 1–5 x 1–5
Leg Curls (2 legs)	2–4 x 4–6
Bent-Leg Dead Lift with Dumbbell	1–3 x 4–6
Two-Arm Dumbbell Lateral Raise	1–3 x 4–6
Two-Arm Bent Lateral Raise	2–4 x 4–6
Seated Cable Row	2–4 x 4–6
Two-Arm Lat Pull Down	2–4 x 4–6
Dumbbell Shrugs	1–3 x 4–6
Deviation	1–3 x 6–8
Gripper	1–3 x 6–8
Lying Twist	1–3 x 10–20
Seated Twist	1–3 x 10–20

Clean dead lift, clean pull, squat, and bench press. What does 50%–85% x 1–3 x 1–5 mean during the preseason? Several types of workouts can come from this type of prescription. The sets and repetitions can vary depending on how the athlete feels:

- 50% x 3 x 5
- 70% x 3 x 3
- 85% x 3 x 1–5
- 65% x 1–5, 75% x 1–5, 85% x 1–5

In theory, it is nice to have laid out daily training plans that appear to fit the spring training schedule (e.g., games, practice, travel, etc.), but the reality is that sometimes the player is just not up to what is planned for the day. So, rather than not train at all, which could be an alternative, there have to be other choices.

Supplemental lifts: Low volume is the key during this time of year for several reasons:

1. To facilitate the handling of moderate to heavy weight

2. To decrease the soreness that usually occurs with high repetitions

3. To eliminate the chance of increasing fatigue levels

Gripping and rotational exercises have to be implemented with caution. An increase in swinging and throwing could lead to overtraining, resulting in wrist and forearm injury as well as lower-back issues. One set with all-out effort and maximum resistance might be all that is necessary following a busy day on the field.

	IN-SEASON—FIELDERS (sets x reps)	
Month	**Core Lifts (Clean dead lift, clean pull, bench press, squat, one-leg squat)**	**Supplemental Lifts**
April	60%–85% x 3–5 x 5	3–5 x 8
May	60%–85% x 3–5 x 5	3–5 x 5
June	60%–92.5% x 3–5 x 3	3–5 x 8
July	60%–92.5% x 3–5 x 3	3–5 x 5
August	60%–100% x 3–5 x 1–2	3–5 x 8
September	60%–100% x 3–5 x 1–2	3–5 x 5

The above format is a general template that can be followed throughout the professional season. Due to the long, tiring year, the percentages listed for the core lifts are only an estimation of the work performed and not exact poundage. In other words, one assumes that five repetitions with the heaviest weight possible is an 85% effort. Why not exact poundage similar to the off-season and preseason programs? Because unlike the other phases of the year, the in-season's grueling schedule of games and travel makes it difficult to predict the strength levels of the athlete. That being said, it makes more sense to adjust the weight to fit the repetition range and the player's energy level. As a result, using a set of five repetitions as the example, an athlete may not be able to train with his personal best poundage, but it will be his best maximum effort. September is further illustration of the in-season training philosophy in which the athlete is asked to use maximum effort for one repetition, and that is not likely to be, after six months of baseball, his personal best poundage.

Sets and repetitions for the supplemental lifts vary little over the course of the season. Again, the lower repetition range prevents on-the-field fatigue caused by weight training while still training in a repetition zone best suited for strength.

As recovery and rest are critical for performance over a six-month period, lighter than normal weights must be used at intervals during the season. The "three up, one down" method is one of several ways to achieve this. By training with maximum weights (the upper end of the percentage range) for three consecutive weeks, and in the fourth week using lighter weights (the lower end of the percentage range), the athlete has a physical and mental break from training without taking an entire week off:

EXAMPLE: APRIL (sets x reps)		
WEEK	CORE LIFTS	SUPPLEMENTAL LIFTS
Week 1	75% x 4 x 5	100% intensity 3 x 8
Week 2	80% x 3 x 5	100% intensity 4 x 8
Week 3	85% x 3 x 4	100% intensity 4 x 8
Week 4	65% x 3 x 3	60% intensity 3 x 8

FIVE-DAY SCHEDULE

DAY ONE • *Total body power (clean dead lift, clean pull), hamstrings/lower back, forearms/grip exercises.*

Clean pull

Leg curls

Bent-leg dead lift with dumbbell

DAY TWO • *Chest, abdominals/rotational exercises.*

Bench press

Incline barbell bench press

Three-way chop

Lying twist

DAY THREE • *Shoulders/trapezius, forearms/grip exercises.*

Two-arm dumbbell lateral raise

One-arm bent lateral raise with cable

Dumbbell shrugs

DAY FOUR • *Latissimus/rhomboids exercises.*

Dumbbell row

One-arm lat pull down

Seated row

DAY FIVE • *Quadriceps, abdominals/rotational exercises.*

Squat or one-leg squat
Deviation
Gripper

After a long day at the ballpark (arriving at the field by noon for a 7 P.M. game), the last thing a player wants to do is attack a 45–60 minute weight training session at 11 P.M.! Shorter, intense workouts ranging from 10–30 minutes are the best bet for consistent work throughout the season. Hard and heavy!

IN-SEASON—STARTING PITCHERS

DAY ONE	Pitch
DAY TWO	Upper body weight training*
DAY THREE	Lower body weight training*
DAY FOUR	No weight training
DAY FIVE	No weight training
DAY SIX	Pitch

* The exercises, sets, and repetitions will be the same as illustrated in the fielder's program.

The in-season is really the only time when special programming is in effect for starting pitchers. Traditionally, a five-day rotation is employed, which puts the pitcher on the mound every five days. With the proposed schedule, the pitcher will lift two times per "turn," with the preference of which half of the body he trains on days two and three. The rationale behind this type of program is simple: resting the day after pitching is the logical choice, but with only four days before the next start, a full day of inactivity is not suitable. So it makes sense to weight train the furthest away from his next start by utilizing days two and three, giving him two full days of recovery before the next outing.

PROFESSIONAL WEIGHT TRAINING SUMMARY

Aside from first-time lifters, all of the programs are essentially the same. The key in professional sports is injury prevention, not development. In other words, increasing strength and power is secondary to keeping the players on the field.

Besides, common sense tells us that if these athletes needed further development, they would not be in the Big Leagues. Granted, some players drafted out of high school and players only one or two years out of college may need some added development. But if you expected something complex, or to use the exaggerated marketing term "cutting edge," you would be misinformed and disappointed. What you see at the professional level is solid training principles employed by learned practitioners in concert with the team's athletic trainer and physicians—the most effective method.

Creating a training program is the easy part—the real coaching comes with daily supervision from February to (hopefully) October: knowing when to decrease weight, modify or substitute exercises, adjust repetitions and sets, and sometimes switch the workout days—on the spot. This type of practice can only be done in the course of daily supervision and observation of the athlete; in other words, in full-time coaching. This is why it is careless, if not make-believe, to suggest a program can be implemented without examining the professional baseball player's six-month daily activity (including game observation) and without consulting with a team's sports medicine staff.

Appendix D

Summary of Weight Training Programs

The most important theme to all the training programs is that the "basics" work the best. The fundamental methods and theories, contrary to what some coaches will have you believe, have always outperformed the latest training "innovations," and they always will.

This book would need to be an encyclopedia to list every basic barbell and dumbbell exercise. Instead, we have given you a few basic movements and, more importantly, have listed the key musculature to be trained. Your creativity and knowledge will lead to programs that could essentially have an entirely different menu of exercises, yet accomplish the same objectives.

Additionally, the younger and less experienced an athlete is, the less complicated his program needs to be. The group of athletes and coaches that violate this philosophy the most are the group that stands to benefit the most from elementary training—the high school–aged group. There is little scientific support (if any) for high school athletes to be involved in weight training programs with lengthy menus and complicated exercises that last ninety minutes or longer. One could argue that sixty minutes is too much! It is not too mind-boggling to think that a young athlete could bench press, squat, and clean dead lift for four years and make more physical progress than those performing 2–3 times as many exercises. Point made. In review, there should be a clear progression, basic to complex, from the high school years to the college years and from the college years to the professional ranks.

Lastly, mimicry may be the sincerest form of flattery, but in the world of strength and conditioning, mimicry can keep athletes from realizing their physical potential or, even worse, result in injury. The world champions, collegiate national powers, and even the country's finest high school teams have programs that are tailored to their specific situations:

- Training experience of the athlete
- Size of the training facility
- Equipment inventory
- Number of available supervisors
- Coaching expertise
- Frequency and duration limitations (length of training sessions and how many per week)

Implementing clean pulls without expertise in the Olympic weightlifting movements; condensing a three-day plan into two days; training forty athletes in a facility that can only safely accommodate twenty-five; using professional or college programs at the high school level—these are all ways to hinder an athlete's development.

Frankly, just because it works for someone else does not mean it will work for you. Programs should be designed based on the needs of the athletes who are going to use it, the facility where they are going to train, and the coaches who are going to coach them.

The strongest men in the world started with, and for the most part have stayed with, the simplest of movements to get strong.

References

Aagaard, P. "Creatine Supplementation Augments the Increase in Satellite Cell and Myonuclei Number in Human Skeletal Muscle Induced by Strength Training." *J Physiol.* (2006).

Acheson, K.J., G. Gremaud, I. Meirim, et al. "Metabolic Effects of Caffeine in Humans: Lipid Oxidation or Futile Cycling?" *Am J Clin Nutr* 79. (2004): 40–46.

Antonio, J., et al. "Effects of Exercise Training and Amino-acid Supplementation on Body Composition and Physical Performance in Untrained Women." *Nutrition.* 16:11–12 (2000): 1043–1046.

Arciero, P.J., C.L. Bougopoulos, B.C. Nindl, et al. "Influence of Age on the Thermic Response to Caffeine in Women." *Metabolism.* 49 (2000): 101–107.

Arciero, P.J., A.W. Gardner, J. Calles-Escandon, et al. "Effects of Caffeine Ingestion on NE Kinetics, Fat Oxidation, and Energy Expenditure in Younger and Older Men." *Am J Physiol.* 268 (1995): E1192–E1198.

Armstrong, L.E. "Caffeine, Body Fluid-Electrolyte Balance, and Exercise Performance." *Int J Sport Nutr Exerc Metab.* 12:2 (2002): 189–206.

Astrup, A., S. Toubro, S. Cannon, et al. "Caffeine: A Double-blind, Placebo-controlled Study of Its Thermogenic, Metabolic, and Cardiovascular Effects in Healthy Volunteers." *Am J Clin Nutr.* 51 (1990): 759–767.

Bermon, S., P. Venembre, C. Sachet, et al. "Effects of Creatine Monohydrate Ingestion in Sedentary and Weight-trained Older Adults." *Acta Physiol Scand.* 164 (1998): 147–155.

Bird, S.P., K.M. Tarpenning, and F.E. Marino. "Independent and Combined Effects of Liquid Carbohydrate/Essential Amino Acid Ingestion on Hormonal and Muscular Adaptations Following Resistance Training in Untrained Men." *Eur J Appl Physiol.* (2006): 1–14.

Bracco, D., J.M. Ferrarra, M.J. Arnaud, et al. "Effects of Caffeine on Energy Metabolism, Heart Rate, and Methylxanthine Metabolism in Lean and Obese Women." *Am J Physiol.* 269 (1995): E671–E678.

Burke, D.G., P.D. Chilibeck, K.S. Davidson, et al. "The Effect of Whey Protein Supplementation With and Without Creatine Monohydrate Combined with Resistance Training on Lean Tissue Mass and Muscle Strength." *Int J Sport Nutr Exerc Metab.* 11 (2001): 349–364.

Casey, A., et al. "Creatine Ingestion Favorably Affects Performance and Muscle Metabolism During Maximal Exercise in Humans." *Am J Physiol.* 271:1 Part 1 (1996): E31–E37.

Cavin, C., D. Holzhaeuser, G. Scharf, et al. "Cafestol and Kahweol, Two Coffee-specific Diterpenes with Anticarcinogenic Activity." *Food Chem Toxicol.* 40:8 (2002): 1155–1163.

Cheung, W.T., C.M. Lee, and T.B. Ng. "Potentiation of the Anti-lipolytic Effect of 2-Chloroadenosine after Chronic Caffeine Treatment." *Pharmacology.* 36 (1988): 331–339.

Crowe, M.J., J.N. Weatherson, and B.F. Bowden. "Effects of Dietary Leucine Supplementation on Exercise Performance." *Eur J Appl Physiol.* (2005): 1–9.

Dulloo, A.G., C.A. Geissler, T. Horton, et al. "Normal Caffeine Consumption: Influence on Thermogenesis and Daily Energy Expenditure in Lean and Post-obese Human Volunteers." *Am J Clin Nutr.* 49 (1989): 44–50.

Earnest, C.P., P.G. Snell, R. Rodriguez, et al. "The Effect of Creatine Monohydrate Ingestion on Anaerobic Power Indices, Muscular Strength and Body Composition." *Acta Physiol Scand.* 153 (1995): 207–209.

Grandjean, A.C., et al. "The Effect of Caffeinated, Non-caffeinated, Caloric and Non-caloric Beverages on Hydration." *J Am Coll Nutr.* 19:5 (2000): 591–600.

Greenhaff, P.L., A. Casey, A.H. Short, et al. "Influence of Oral Creatine Supplementation of Muscle Torque During Repeated Bouts of Maximal Voluntary Exercise in Man." *Clin Sci (Lond).* 84 (1993): 565–571.

Greenwood, M., et al. "Creatine Supplementation Patterns and Perceived Effects in Select Division I Collegiate Athletes." *Clin J Sport Med.* 10:3 (2000): 191–194.

Greenwood, M., et al. "Cramping and Injury Incidence in Collegiate Football Players are Reduced by Creatine Supplementation." *J Athl Train.* 38:3 (2003): 216–219.

Greenwood, M., et al. "Creatine Supplementation During College Football Training Does Not Increase the Incidence of Cramping or Injury." *Mol Cell Biochem.* 244:1–2 (2003): 83–88.

Harris, R.C., et al. "The Absorption of Orally Supplied Beta-alanine and Its Effect on Muscle Carnosine Synthesis in Human Vastus Lateralis." *Amino Acids.* 30:3 (2006): 279–289.

Hetzler, R.K., R.G. Knowlton, S.M. Somani, et al. "Effect of Paraxanthine on FFA Mobilization after Intravenous Caffeine Administration in Humans." *J Appl Physiol.* 68 (1990): 44–47.

Hill, C.A., et al. "Influence of Beta-alanine Supplementation on Skeletal Muscle Carnosine Concentrations and High-intensity Cycling Capacity." *Amino Acids.* (2006).

Izawa, T., E. Koshimizu, T. Komabayashi, et al. ["Effects of Ca2+ and Calmodulin Inhibitors on Lipolysis Induced by Epinephrine, Norepinephrine, Caffeine and ACTH in Rat Epididymal Adipose Tissue."] *Nippon Seirigaku Zasshi.* 45 (1983): 36–44.

Jiang, M., K. Kameda, L.K. Han, et al. "Isolation of Lipolytic Substances Caffeine and 1,7-Dimethylxanthine from the Stem and Rhizome of *Sinomenium actum.*" *Planta Med.* 64 (1998): 375–377.

Jordan, S.J., D.M. Purdie, A.C. Green, et al. "Coffee, Tea and Caffeine and Risk of Epithelial Ovarian Cancer." *Cancer Causes Control.* 15:4 (2004): 359–365.

Karlson, E.W., L.A. Mandl, G.N. Aweh, et al. "Coffee Consumption and Risk of Rheumatoid Arthritis." *Arthritis Rheum.* 48:11 (2003): 3055–3060.

Kleemola, P., P. Jousilahti, P. Pietinen, et al. "Coffee Consumption and the Risk of Coronary Heart Disease and Death." *Arch Intern Med.* 160:22 (2000): 3393–3400.

Koopman, R., et al. "Combined Ingestion of Protein and Free Leucine with Carbohydrate Increases Postexercise Muscle Protein Synthesis in Vivo in Male Subjects." *Am J Physiol Endocrinol Metab.* 288:4 (2005): E645–E653.

Koot, P., and P. Deurenberg. "Comparison of Changes in Energy Expenditure and Body Temperatures After Caffeine Consumption." *Ann Nutr Metab.* 39 (1995): 135–142.

Kraemer, W.J., and J.S. Volek. "Creatine Supplementation: Its Role in Human Performance." *Clin Sports Med.* 18:3 (1999): 651–666, ix.

Kreider, R.B., et al. "Long-term Creatine Supplementation Does Not Significantly Affect Clinical Markers of Health in Athletes." *Mol Cell Biochem.* 244:1–2 (2003): 95–104.

Lang, C.H. "Elevated Plasma Free Fatty Acids Decrease Basal Protein Synthesis but Not the Anabolic Effect of Leucine in Skeletal Muscle." *Am J Physiol Endocrinol Metab.* (2006).

Lee, S.Y., and K.C. Kim. "Effect of Beta-alanine Administration on Carbon Tetrachloride-induced Acute Hepatotoxicity." *Amino Acids.* (2006).

Michaud, D.S., E. Giovannucci, W.C. Willett, et al. "Coffee and Alcohol Consumption and the Risk of Pancreatic Cancer in Two Prospective United States Cohorts." *Cancer Epidemiol Biomarkers Prev.* 10:5 (2001): 429–437.

Michels, K.B., L. Holmberg, L. Bergkvist, et al. "Coffee, Tea, and Caffeine Consumption and Breast Cancer Incidence in a Cohort of Swedish Women." *Ann Epidemiol.* 12:1 (2002): 21–26.

Mori, H., K. Kawabata, K. Matsunaga, et al. "Chemopreventive Effects of Coffee Bean and Rice Constituents on Colorectal Carcinogenesis." *Biofactors.* 12:1–4 (2000): 101–105.

Morton, C., A.L. Klatsky, and N. Udaltsova. "Smoking, Coffee, and Pancreatitis." *Am J Gastroenterol.* 99:4 (2004): 731–738.

Narod, S.A., S. De Sanjose, and C. Victora. "Coffee During Pregnancy: A Reproductive Hazard?" *Am J Obstet Gynecol.* 164:4 (1991): 1109–1114.

Norton, L.E., and D.K. Layman. "Leucine Regulates Translation Initiation of Protein Synthesis in Skeletal Muscle After Exercise." *J Nutr.* 136:2 (2006): 533S–537S.

Poehlman, E.T., J.P. Despres, H. Bessette, et al. "Influence of Caffeine on the Resting Metabolic Rate of Exercise-trained and Inactive Subjects." *Med Sci Sports Exerc.* 17 (1985): 689–694.

Poortmans, J.R., and M. Francaux. "Adverse Effects of Creatine Supplementation: Fact or Fiction?" *Sports Med.* 30:3 (2000): 155–170.

Poortmans, J.R., and M. Francaux. "Long-term Oral Creatine Supplementation Does Not Impair Renal Function in Healthy Athletes." *Med Sci Sports Exerc.* 31 (1999): 1108–1110.

Powers, M.E., B.L. Arnold, A.L. Weltman, et al. "Creatine Supplementation Increases Total Body Water Without Altering Fluid Distribution." *J Athl Train.* 38 (2003): 44–50.

Ryu, S., S.K. Choi, S.S. Joung, et al. "Caffeine as a Lipolytic Food Component Increases Endurance Performance in Rats and Athletes." *J Nutr Sci Vitaminol (Tokyo).* 47 (2001): 139–146.

Sakamoto, W., J. Nishihira, K. Fujie, et al. "Coffee and Fitness-coffee Suppresses Lipopolysaccharide-induced Liver Injury in Rats." *J Nutr Sci Vitaminol (Tokyo).* 46:6 (2000): 316–320.

Salazar-Martinez, E., W.C. Willett, A. Ascherio, et al. "Coffee Consumption and Risk for Type 2 Diabetes Mellitus." *Ann Intern Med.* 140:1 (2004): 1–8.

Steenge, G.R., P. Verhoef, and P.L. Greenhaff. "The Effect of Creatine and Resistance Training on Plasma Homocysteine Concentration in Healthy Volunteers." *Arch Intern Med.* 161:11 (2001): 1455–1456.

Tarnopolsky, M.A., and M.F. Beal. "Potential for Creatine and Other Therapies Targeting Cellular Energy Dysfunction in Neurological Disorders." *Ann Neurol.* 49:5 (2001): 561–574.

Tarnopolsky, M.A., and D.P. MacLennan. "Creatine Monohydrate Supplementation Enhances High-intensity Exercise Performance in Males and Females." *Int J Sport Nutr Exerc Metab.* 10 (2000): 452–463.

Tarnopolsky, M.A., G. Parise, N.J. Yardley, et al. "Creatine-Dextrose and Protein-Dextrose Induce Similar Strength Gains During Training." *Med Sci Sports Exerc.* 33 (2001): 2044–2052.

Tavani, A., M. Bertuzzi, R. Talamini, et al. "Coffee and Tea Intake and Risk of Oral, Pharyngeal and Esophageal Cancer." *Oral Oncol.* 39:7 (2003): 695–700.

Urbanski, R.L., W.J. Vincent, and B.B. Yaspelkis 3rd. "Creatine Supplementation Differentially Affects Maximal Isometric Strength and Time to Fatigue in Large and Small Muscle Groups." *Int J Sport Nutr.* 9:2 (1999): 136–145.

Volek, J.S., et al. "Performance and Muscle Fiber Adaptations to Creatine Supplementation and Heavy Resistance Training." *Med Sci Sports Exerc.* 31:8 (1999): 1147–1156.

Volek, J.S., W.J. Kraemer, J.A. Bush, et al. "Creatine Supplementation Enhances Muscular Performance During High-intensity Resistance Exercise." *J Am Diet Assoc.* 97 (1997): 765–770.

Volek, J.S., S.A. Mazzetti, W.B. Farquhar, et al. "Physiological Responses to Short-term Exercise in the Heat after Creatine Loading." *Med Sci Sports Exerc.* 33 (2001): 1101–1108.

Volek, J.S., and E.S. Rawson. "Scientific Basis and Practical Aspects of Creatine Supplementation for Athletes." *Nutrition.* 20 (2004): 609–614.

Willoughby, D.S., and J. Rosene. "Effects of Oral Creatine and Resistance Training on Myosin Heavy Chain Expression." *Med Sci Sports Exerc.* 33:10 (2001): 1674–1681.

Willoughby, D.S., J.R. Stout, and C.D. Wilborn. "Effects of Resistance Training and Protein Plus Amino Acid Supplementation on Muscle Anabolism, Mass, and Strength." *Amino Acids.* (2006).

Willoughby, D.S., and J.M. Rosene. "Effects of Oral Creatine and Resistance Training on Myogenic Regulatory Factor Expression." *Med Sci Sports Exerc.* 35 (2003): 923–929.

Zahorska-Markiewicz, B. ["Does Post-caffeine Increase in Thermogenesis Facilitate the Treatment of Obesity?"]. *Pol Tyg Lek.* 35 (1980): 697–699.

Zhang, Y., and J.N. Wells. "The Effects of Chronic Caffeine Administration on Peripheral Adenosine Receptors." *J Pharmacol Exp Ther.* 254 (1990): 757–763.

Ziegenfuss, T.N., et al. "Effect of Creatine Loading on Anaerobic Performance and Skeletal Muscle Volume in NCAA Division I Athletes." *Nutrition.* 18:5 (2002): 397–402.

Zoeller, R.F., J.R. Stout, J.A. O'Kroy, et al. "Effects of 28 Days of Beta-alanine and Creatine Monohydrate Supplementation on Aerobic Power, Ventilatory and Lactate Thresholds, and Time to Exhaustion." *Amino Acids.* (2006).

Index

About the Authors

Bob Alejo is considered one of the world's leading experts on strength and conditioning for baseball. As strength and conditioning director at U.C. Santa Barbara since 2005, Bob brings nearly twenty-five years of unmatched experience training athletes. Bob was also the conditioning coach for the Oakland Athletics baseball team from 1993 to 2001, and from 1984 to 1993 trained and supervised men's and women's teams at the University of California, at Los Angeles. He is a member of the National Strength and Conditioning Association, American College of Sports Medicine, International Society of Sports Nutrition, and is a Certified Strength and Conditioning Specialist as well as a Level-I Weightlifting Federation coach.

Jose Antonio, Ph.D., CSCS, FACSM, FISSN, is the chief executive officer of the International Society of Sports Nutrition (ISSN; www.theissn.org) and one of its cofounders. Dr. Antonio earned his Ph.D. from the University of Texas Southwestern Medical Center, in Dallas, in the area of skeletal muscle plasticity. He also completed a post-doctoral fellowship in endocrinology and metabolism. His latest book project is the *Essentials of Sports Nutrition and Supplements* (Humana Press, expected publication 2008). For more information: www.JoseAntonioPhD.com.

Bill Campbell, Ph.D., CSCS, FISSN, is an assistant professor at the University of South Florida and is the director of the Exercise and Performance Nutrition Laboratory. His primary research focuses on sports nutrition and skeletal muscle physiology. He has published more than fifty research papers and abstracts in the realm of sports nutrition and exercise metabolism. In addition, he is currently the elected secretary for the International Society of Sports Nutrition, a Fellow of ISSN, and is a Certified Strength and Conditioning Specialist.